PRAISE FOR *HIGH-OCTANE BRAIN*

"Although not everyone thinks about the future, in the life of an Olympic athlete we are always looking to the future, sometimes even four years ahead. Our brain and bodies now and in the future are our best tools, and when they don't work 100 percent we are in trouble. If we just treat our brain and body with the proper care, we may outlive our projected time frames. Given my mom had dementia and passed away in 2004 at the age of 86, I hope I can outlive her and be healthy at the time of my passing. Michelle shares with you how to take great care of your brain now and in the future, not just to lower the risk of Alzheimer's, but for better overall health and well-being!"

—**Bonnie Blair,** five-time Olympic gold medalist

"Dr. Braun has written a life-changer, a life-enhancer. In clear, commonsense language with scientific facts, she is proving there is finally a way to fight Alzheimer's. Now [there is] hope where there was none."

—**Martin J. Schreiber,** former governor of Wisconsin and author of *My Two Elaines: Learning, Coping, and Surviving as an Alzheimer's Caregiver*

"Dr. Michelle Braun is at the forefront of the exciting and promising field of 'brain health,' and her new book, *High-Octane Brain*, empowers us all to steer our own aging path using a simple five-step program designed to engage brain health promoting behaviors to reduce dementia risk. Through a mixture of expert interviews, case examples, and practical suggestions, Braun uses her remarkable insights and crystal-clear writing style to convincingly argue that healthy aging is within our reach if we take the opportunity we all have to make healthy lifestyle choices. Written in a way that is inspiring to both lay and professional audiences, *High-Octane Brain* fills the tank with simple tools that allow users to implement her program and to measure progress. It is a 'must have' for those of us who work with aging populations, and those of us who want to invest in a more active, engaged, and healthy future for ourselves."

—**Russell M. Bauer, PhD, ABPP,** Preeminence Term Professor, University of Florida; Director, Brain Rehabilitation Research Center of Excellence, Malcom Randall Veterans' Affairs Medical Center

"An emerging field of neuroscience points to the importance of a healthy lifestyle in reducing the risk of Alzheimer's. . . . Dr. Michelle Braun illustrates in a clear and concise style strategies to maximize brain health and stave off Alzheimer's. Unlike other brain-wellness publications, this book is based on solid scientific evidence, amply documented in the different chapters dealing with nutrition, physical activity, cognitive stimulation, stress reduction and sleep. At the same time, the material is brought to life through interviews with experts, case illustrations, summary tables and takeaway points that make this book an engaging read for the general public. In a time when there are still no pharmacological cures for Alzheimer's, this book shows us a path towards healthy brain aging: a book invaluable not only to the clinician, but to all of us aiming to enhance our brain health and quality of life in our later years."

—Piero G. Antuono, MD, Professor of Neurology and Biophysics,
Medical College of Wisconsin; Member, Medical and Scientific
Advisory Panel, Alzheimer's Disease International

"Medical science has lessened the impact of many previously fatal diseases, but alas, not Alzheimer's, which threatens to overwhelm our health and long-term care systems and devastate more and more families. In the face of this crisis, Dr. Michelle Braun offers us a way in our everyday lives to confront Alzheimer's head-on, and cheers us on into believing we can succeed. In the process, she deftly straddles the complex worlds of neuroanatomy and brain science, condenses it all into concise lifestyle advice, and presents it in steps that are engaging, doable, and fun. Readers that follow her game plan will live much more enjoyable lives . . . not to mention the three-pound blob of tissue in your skull that makes you who you are will thank you profusely!"

—Tom Hlavacek, Retired Executive Director,
Alzheimer's Association Southeastern Wisconsin Chapter

High-Octane Brain

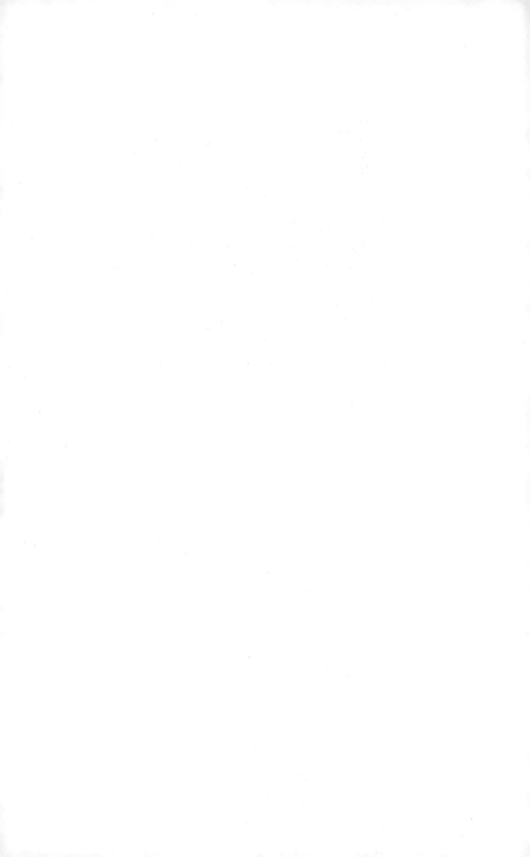

High-Octane Brain

5 SCIENCE-BASED STEPS
TO SHARPEN YOUR MEMORY AND
REDUCE YOUR RISK OF ALZHEIMER'S

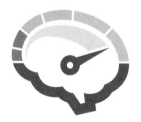

Dr. Michelle Braun
Foreword by Dr. Karen Postal

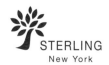

STERLING
New York

STERLING
New York

An Imprint of Sterling Publishing Co., Inc.
1166 Avenue of the Americas
New York, NY 10036

ISBN 978-1-4549-3778-4

Distributed in Canada by Sterling Publishing Co., Inc.
c/o Canadian Manda Group, 664 Annette Street
Toronto, Ontario M6S 2C8, Canada
Distributed in the United Kingdom by GMC Distribution Services
Castle Place, 166 High Street, Lewes, East Sussex BN7 1XU, England
Distributed in Australia by NewSouth Books
University of New South Wales, Sydney, NSW 2052, Australia

For information about custom editions, special sales, and premium and
corporate purchases, please contact Sterling Special Sales at 800-805-5489 or
specialsales@sterlingpublishing.com.

Manufactured in Canada

2 4 6 8 10 9 7 5 3 1

sterlingpublishing.com

Cover design by Igor Satanovsky
Interior design by Gavin C. Motnyk

Picture Credits - see page 269

Dedication

To Adam and Halle: the inspiration for my High-Octane Brain journey.

Contents

List of Figures and Tables. ix

Foreword:

    Dr. Karen Postal, Harvard Medical School. xi

Preface. xv

Introduction: Your Future Self 1

PART I

THE NEW GAME-CHANGING RULES OF BRAIN AGING

  1. The High-Octane Brain Revolution. 8

  2. The Journey Begins. 29

  3. A Fresh Start: How to Maximize Your Brain Health 41

PART II

5 STEPS TO A HIGH-OCTANE BRAIN:

THE EXCELS METHOD

  4. Step 1: **EX**ercise Is the X-Factor 58

  5. Step 2: **C**onsume Healthy Food 81

  6. Step 3: **E**ngage and Learn 107

  7. Step 4: **L**ower Stress and Boost Well-Being. 129

  8. Step 5: **S**leep for Better Brain Power. 150

PART III
HIGH-OCTANE BRAIN ROLE MODELS

9. Meet Your Brain Health Success Squad:
High-Octane Brain Role Models Ages 44 to 83 168

10. Meet Your Brain Health Hall of Famers:
High-Octane Brain Role Models Ages 91 to 103 188

Coda: Meredith and Lou: Closing the Circle 205

Acknowledgments 212

Appendix I

How to Use the High-Octane Brain Tracker 214

High-Octane Action Plan Form 216

High-Octane Tracker 219

Appendix II

Dr. Melanie Chandler on Treatment of Mild Cognitive Impairment 231

Notes 241

Brain Health Expert Contributors 257

Index 260

Picture Credits 269

About the Author and Foreword Author 270

List of Figures and Tables

FIGURES

Fig. 1: Three Possible Brain Health Trajectories for Each Individual...... 10

Fig. 2: Three-Path Choice Regarding Your Future Brain Health......... 51

Fig. 3: Hippocampal Growth After Cardiovascular Exercise............. 63

Fig. 4: High-Octane Tracker Exercise (Example)...................... 78

Fig. 5: Brain Blip 1: Forgetting the Name of Someone You Just Met 121

Fig. 6: Brain Blip 2: Misplacing Objects.............................. 122

Fig. 7: Brain Blip 4: Word-Finding Difficulties........................ 124

TABLES

Bonus Benefits to Physical Activity 71

Movement Matrix 72

Nutrients and Physiology 97

MIND Diet Component Servings and Scoring (Example) 100

Foreword

I f there was a pill that could reduce your chances of developing Alzheimer's disease by 50 percent, would you take it? What if the only side effects of the pill were better fitness, more energy, and greater emotional health? What if the pill was free? Over the last two decades, there has been a grim string of failures to cure Alzheimer's disease with an actual pill. However, during that time compelling research has demonstrated that the same lifestyle factors associated with heart health also result in brain health. Not just one study supports this finding but hundreds of them, and they all converge on the same idea: successful brain aging is not about luck and is not random. We have the ability to shape the health of our brains. How many people know, for example, that when we exercise, we trigger neurogenesis (the birth of new brain cells) in the memory centers of our brains? How many know what we eat, how much we sleep and exercise, and our level of intellectual curiosity and social engagement also have a direct, positive impact on maintaining a healthy brain throughout the life span?

Why hasn't this research become part of mainstream consciousness? We have certainly bought into the idea that infants' brains are positively shaped by nutrition, exercise, and a stimulating environment. At the first signs of pregnancy, parents and grandparents invest in toys, music, and devices that are said to stimulate neural connections and improve thinking. We hang black-and-white mobiles over cribs to stimulate babies' vision. We play Mozart in the nursery. We choose formula with the omega-3 fatty acid DHA to promote brain cell myelination.

Maybe it's the Freudian notion that personalities are set by early childhood that dampens a similar enthusiasm for optimizing brain function beyond toddlerhood—for the public and researchers alike. Even as more and more neuroscience research demonstrates that our brains continue to be shaped by diet, exercise, and stimulating environments well into our eighties and nineties, the general public has not become concerned with optimizing brain function and memory in adulthood and late life.

The same thing goes for the field of neuroscience. Instead, we clinicians and researchers spend most of our energy measuring cognitive decline and disease. For years we focused on large populations of aging individuals who, when viewed as a whole, have brains that slowly atrophy and thinking abilities that slip with every passing decade. But what if we looked at the same data in another way? What if we searched for the individuals who remain mentally sharp, who don't show the typical brain atrophy and thinking declines over time? What's different about these successful agers? The resounding answer is lifestyle factors. As this data on brain health piles up, burgeoning ranks of neuropsychologists and neuroscientists are shifting our attention. Rather than focusing solely on diagnosing and treating dementia syndromes, why don't we help people think better by optimizing brain health throughout their lives?

Dr. Michelle Braun is in the forefront of this movement. In my own work with Alzheimer's patients, along with my research on improving the ways we share neuroscience with the general public, I recognize how profoundly important it is to get the most current information on brain health out in a vivid, accessible way. I remember watching in awe when Michelle appeared on a PBS special in which her unique mix of personal warmth, passion, and intellectual clarity was on full display as she discussed brain health. Her gift of explaining neuroscience in an accessible, practical, and affirming way is what earned her the Practitioner of the Year Award from the Alzheimer's Association of Southeastern Wisconsin in 2008 and what makes her *Psychology Today* blog on brain health so popular. I have known Michelle for years as a leader in the field of neuropsychology, and so when she told me that she was writing a book on brain health for a general audience, I broke out in a huge smile. Who better to advance the conversation about improving brain health than a neuropsychologist who is serious about presenting accurate, research-based information in an engaging and passionate way? I'm delighted to say that *High-Octane Brain* is everything I hoped it would be when Michelle first told me about the idea: a profoundly hopeful, evidence-based road map to healthy brain aging.

—Karen Postal, PhD, ABPP
Harvard Medical School

Preface

Welcome! This book offers science-based guidance and a five-step tracking system to optimize brain health and memory and significantly decrease the risk of developing Alzheimer's disease. The information presented here is intended to encourage and support the pursuit of optimal brain health, but it is not designed to substitute for medical advice and evaluation. Please consult with your healthcare provider before making any changes that are based on what you learn in this book. Unless otherwise noted, I use the term "Alzheimer's" to refer to the 99 percent of cases of Alzheimer's-related dementia that do not have a genetic cause, not to the 1 percent of cases of genetically caused familial-onset Alzheimer's.

Note that the names, identifying details, and specific issues of the two clients in the book—Meredith and Lou—have been changed to protect their privacy. The book also includes interviews with eight leading experts who have profoundly advanced our understanding of neuroscience and brain health. However, since none of the experts reviewed any material except their own interviews, their participation does not serve as an endorsement of this book.

Finally, you will meet nine inspiring High-Octane Brain role models who graciously agreed to share their names and life stories so that you could learn how they cultivated optimal brain health. Their stories—and the science behind the High-Octane Brain program in this book—demonstrate that the journey of brain health is rich and unexpectedly rewarding and touches all corners of our lives.

Introduction

Your Future Self

Most of us think about our brain in the present tense. We may experience its sluggishness when we don't sleep enough or its occasional difficulty remembering the name of a person we just met or the reason we walked into a room. Sometimes we think about our brain in retrospect, wistfully comparing it to what it was years ago. But most of us don't think about our future brain. It could be because we don't know that we are literally shaping our future brain with every behavior in which we engage (or don't engage) right now. We may not realize that optimizing our future brain is not only possible but the most powerful strategy we have to sharpen our memory, reduce the risk of Alzheimer's, and boost our well-being. Everything we cherish—from our life's work to our engagement with the people and activities we love—is yoked to the health of our future brain. Quite simply, that elegant supercomputer reading this right now is the CEO of all you are, and all you will be. And thankfully, that CEO reports to you.

Over the last several years, the science of brain health and the study of epigenetics (the way our behavior affects the expression of our genes) have converged around a basic hopeful message:

 The lifestyle choices you make today can significantly improve the trajectory of your future brain health regardless of your genetics.

What this means is that wherever you fall on the genetic brain health spectrum—whether you do or don't have a genetic risk for

Alzheimer's—you can improve your future brain health significantly.[1] By extension, you can improve your future relationships, work, passions, and overall well-being.

This does not mean that people who develop Alzheimer's have failed to live a healthy life or are to blame for their illness. Lifestyle factors are only one piece of the Alzheimer's puzzle. However, lifestyle changes are the only proven method we have to reduce the likelihood that Alzheimer's will occur. They are also the only way to delay the start of Alzheimer's symptoms. In fact, as you'll learn in this book, some lifestyle factors have been shown to reduce the risk of Alzheimer's by more than 80 percent,[2] delay the expression of Alzheimer's symptoms by over 10 years,[3] and reduce the amount of Alzheimer's-related cellular changes in the brain.[4]

What Are "Lifestyle Factors"?

Lifestyle factors are modifiable habits that impact health and quality of life. They include diet, exercise, stress management, sleep, and substance use (e.g. alcohol and cigarettes).

The need for this message to reach a widespread audience has reached a fever pitch. A new case of Alzheimer's develops worldwide every 3 seconds[5] and in the United States every 65 seconds.[6] Unfortunately, there is no cure for Alzheimer's, no new medications have been approved since 2003, and several major pharmaceutical companies have exited the Alzheimer's market. In addition, the recent failure of the most promising Alzheimer's drug in years—aducanumab—devastated the Alzheimer's community. In light of the fact that Alzheimer's-related cellular changes can develop 30 years or more before symptoms begin,[7] it has become increasingly clear that we are unlikely to treat it successfully with medication that is administered decades after the disease has taken hold.

Simultaneously, new research has shown an increased risk of Alzheimer's for individuals with a family history of the disease among their parents, siblings, grandparents, cousins, aunts, uncles, and in some cases even more distant relatives,[8] creating an increasing demand for proven information on how to reduce the risk of Alzheimer's and enhance brain health.

In addition to lowering the risk of Alzheimer's, lifestyle factors have been shown to significantly slow the normal age-related cognitive decline that most people experience, sometimes by more than 10 years.[9] Lifestyle factors also help decrease the rate of other common age-related brain changes: problems with word finding and multitasking, memory decline starting in the early thirties,[10] and shrinkage of several key brain regions in late adulthood.[11] This is promising news, especially for the 75 percent of adults who are worried that their brain health will decline in the future and want to do something about it.[12]

Unfortunately, several factors make it difficult to ensure that effective brain health strategies are put into widespread practice. The public often is misled by myths, misinformation, and pseudoscience that encourage people to spend time and money on strategies that are not maximally helpful.[13] Some of those strategies include playing online brain games, taking memory supplements, following restrictive "brain health" diets, getting unnecessary brain scans, and engaging in tasks that are only minimally helpful on their own, such as crosswords. Tragically, ineffective strategies and misconceptions about brain health and Alzheimer's can lead to a false sense of security and years of lost time that otherwise could be spent truly improving brain health.

This book addresses the need for accurate, actionable information by incorporating the strongest science on brain health and Alzheimer's risk reduction into a five-step tracking system that can be completed in just minutes a day. You also will find answers to the following questions as well as many others that often are misunderstood:

- Are my memory problems normal?
- What are the most effective strategies to reduce memory decline and the risk of Alzheimer's?
- Should I take brain health supplements?
- Do brain games work?
- Can I maximize my brain health if I have a family history of memory problems or Alzheimer's?
- How can I boost my memory in minutes?
- What should I eat to optimize brain health?
- What type and duration of exercise are best to reduce the risk of Alzheimer's?
- How can I stay inspired on the journey toward better brain health?

Since 2005, I've shared the science of brain health—and strategies to personalize the brain health journey—via hundreds of "Boost Your Brain" presentations and in neuropsychological evaluations of more than 5,000 clients. As the rate of Alzheimer's and unproven products geared toward preventing it increase exponentially, the need to share this information more broadly has never been more important—and has fueled my passion to write this book.

What Is a High-Octane Brain?

A High-Octane Brain is the optimal brain health trajectory that each of us can achieve: our *personal best* level of brain health. A High-Octane Brain is experienced by individuals with high levels of brain-healthy habits and is associated with the following outcomes:

- A significantly slowed rate of cognitive aging
- Reduced rates of age-related brain shrinkage
- A significantly reduced risk of Alzheimer's
- Delayed expression of Alzheimer's symptoms even if there already are related brain changes or a genetic risk
- Decreased Alzheimer's-related cellular abnormalities in the brain
- Enhanced memory functioning
- Enhanced well-being

THE HIGH-OCTANE BRAIN APPROACH

Anyone who has tried to change his or her exercise, diet, or other ingrained lifestyle habits knows that this is anything but easy. Healthy behaviors tend to be the first casualty of a busy schedule and often take a back seat to the stresses of daily life. Regrettably, the cost of not integrating brain-healthy habits is high not just for ourselves but for our loved ones, our communities, and those we serve. To answer the need for a practical system that we truly can integrate into our lives, this book fuses the best science in brain health (the *what*) with the best science in behavior change and motivational enhancement (the *how*). It strives to unite the head and the heart on a journey that requires both.

This focus on the *what* and the *how* is threaded through each of the exercises, the brain health tracking system, the stories of Meredith and

Lou (two amazing individuals you will follow throughout the book as they integrate brain-healthy habits), and the testimonials of the High-Octane Brain role models. The *what* and the *how* also are incorporated into interviews with brain health experts who graciously share how they integrate brain health habits into their own lives.

 We are on the journey of brain health together, and we will never accomplish it perfectly. But we must keep moving forward because the rewards are too high to forfeit and the cost of not doing so is too great.

Are you ready to elevate your three-pound CEO to High-Octane Brain status? To experience enhanced memory, reduced risk of Alzheimer's, and well-being that comes with it?

Great! Let's begin.

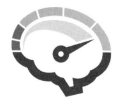

PART I

The New Game-Changing Rules of Brain Aging

"A vision is not just a picture of what could be; it is an appeal to our better selves, a call to become something more."

—Rosabeth Moss Kanter

CHAPTER 1

The High-Octane Brain Revolution

"The best time to plant a tree was twenty years ago.
The second-best time is today."

—CHINESE PROVERB

"The other day, I was in the middle of a conversation, and I knew the exact word I wanted to say but I couldn't think of it. I've also been misplacing my keys more often and forgetting why I walk into a room. All my friends have the same experiences, so I think it's normal. But I'm not sure."

Have you experienced these concerns? I've asked thousands of adults from their teens to their nineties if they can relate to these experiences, and nearly everyone can. Many people chuckle with relief when they learn that their "brain blips" are totally normal. But they're also eager for answers to common questions about brain health and Alzheimer's, including the following:

1. How can I stay mentally sharp as I age?

2. Does _____ really help improve memory? (Fill in the blank with any of the popular techniques that purport to enhance memory, including online brain games, supplements, crosswords, and brain health diets.)

3. What are the strongest science-backed strategies to enhance brain health and reduce the risk of Alzheimer's?

4. When is a memory problem more than a brain blip and a possible harbinger of Alzheimer's?

5. What if Alzheimer's runs in my family? Does it help to try to reduce my risk, or will my genetics win out?

6. How can I make brain health practical and fit it into my busy schedule?

These questions are top of mind for many people—especially if they've known or cared for someone with Alzheimer's disease—and are the subject of this book. Perhaps you have similar concerns about your memory and thinking skills or those of your loved ones. Recent surveys show a widespread fear of Alzheimer's, fueled in part by the prediction that 10 million baby boomers will be diagnosed with the disease. In fact, Americans report fearing Alzheimer's more than any other health condition,[14] and a record 23 million of America's 77 million baby boomers are worried about getting it. In recognition of this trend, the Alzheimer's Association refers to Alzheimer's as "the defining disease of the baby boomers."

Worldwide, 47 million people, including 5.8 million Americans, have been diagnosed with Alzheimer's, and—almost incomprehensibly—this number is projected to nearly triple by 2050.[15] If we could use lifestyle factors to delay the onset of Alzheimer's by even one year, it could lead to 9 million fewer cases by 2050.[16] The good news is that we have powerful proven strategies available right now to reduce the risk of Alzheimer's and/or significantly delay its onset.

A recent review showed that 35 percent of cases of dementia were attributable to a combination of nine mostly behavioral risk factors.[17] Recent cutting-edge clinical trials have also shown a powerful cause-and-effect relationship between healthy lifestyle habits and enhanced brain health. The brain health science behind decreasing the risk of Alzheimer's is so compelling that it has been incorporated into guidelines from several leading national and international organizations, including the Centers for Disease Control,[18] the World Health Organization,[19] the Alzheimer's Association,[20] and the National Academy of Science, Engineering, and Medicine.[21] The need for this information will only continue to grow because the global population of adults age 65 and older is projected to almost double from 2015 to 2050 (from 12 percent to 22 percent).[22]

Adding to the confusion around Alzheimer's, many people don't know there is no direct genetic cause for 99 percent of the cases[23] or that 75 percent of those with Alzheimer's don't have a family history of the disease.[24] The result is that people do not try to adopt lifestyle factors that have been shown to protect against the disease. Even folks not specifically concerned about developing Alzheimer's often wonder what they can do to enhance brain function. They probably recognize the foundational role of brain health in relationships, professional activities, hobbies, and whatever they care about deeply, but they often end up confused about the best way to enhance their brain function.

To put the benefits of a High-Octane Brain into perspective, let's look at the three main brain health trajectories, or paths, we are on at any particular moment that affect our future brain health.

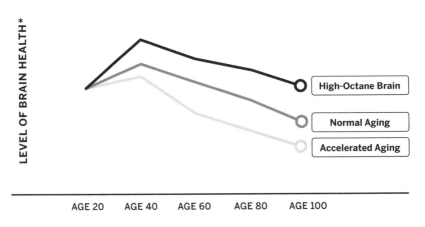

THREE POSSIBLE BRAIN HEALTH TRAJECTORIES
FOR EACH INDIVIDUAL

Figure 1
* = Higher cognitive functioning and brain volume for age

TRAJECTORY 1: NORMAL AGING

The middle line in figure 1 on the opposite page is the trajectory of normal aging, which represents most individuals. This trajectory involves normal age-related declines in brain tissue, brain function, and cognitive functioning. Many people are surprised to learn that cognitive functioning begins to decline at younger ages than expected. For example, on neuropsychological tests (which allow for the precise measurement and tracking of cognitive functioning over time) the average person begins to show declines in spatial visualization and spatial reasoning by the mid-twenties. By the early thirties, declines in memory and reasoning/problem solving are present; and by the mid-thirties, declines in the speed of information processing are evident.[25] Although these declines are initially subtle, they add up with each passing decade and often become more noticeable after age 50.

However, it is important (and encouraging) to note that normal aging also brings cognitive benefits, including increased knowledge of factual information, improved decision making from greater use of wisdom, and improved vocabulary/word knowledge.[26]

Shrinkage (atrophy) of brain tissue typically begins later than declines in cognitive function. For example, shrinkage of the cortex (the outer surface of the brain, responsible for complex information processing) usually begins after age 65,[27] and the hippocampus—one of the most important regions of memory processing in the brain—shrinks in late adulthood at a rate of about 1 to 2 percent per year. There's also progressive age-related shrinkage of several other brain regions.[28] On a normal aging trajectory, there's an average risk of Alzheimer's and/or symptoms of Alzheimer's if related cellular changes are already present.

TRAJECTORY 2: ACCELERATED AGING

The bottom line in the figure represents the trajectory of accelerated aging. This trajectory is defined by an increased decline in memory and other cognitive skills and a significantly increased risk of Alzheimer's. Accelerated aging occurs for a variety of reasons (see chapter 3, pages 45–48), including genetics, health issues, and lifestyle factors.

What Is Alzheimer's?

The term "Alzheimer's" refers to abnormal cellular changes that compromise brain function and often destroy brain tissue. The disease was discovered in 1906 by Dr. Alois Alzheimer after he analyzed the brain tissue of Auguste Deter, a German woman who died at age 55 after exhibiting memory loss and behavioral problems. Dr. Alzheimer identified protein abnormalities that have become the hallmark of the disease named after him—beta-amyloid plaques and neurofibrillary tangles. *Plaques*, which are abnormal clumps of beta-amyloid protein (a naturally occurring protein in the brain), disrupt communication *between* nerve cells, often decades before clinical symptoms begin.

Tangles are formed later in the disease process when *tau*, another naturally occurring brain protein, starts to gather abnormally. In a normal brain, tau helps form the skeleton of neurons (nerve cells). In individuals with Alzheimer's, tau begins to stick to itself and becomes tangled, disrupting communication *within* nerve cells. Alzheimer's also involves other physical changes in the brain, including inflammation, impaired neuronal communication, and a loss of neurons.[29]

"Dementia" is an umbrella term that describes a decline in memory and/or other thinking skills such as language, organizational abilities, decision making, attention, and visual reasoning, among others. With dementia, that decline is beyond what is expected for normal aging, and the condition compromises the ability to carry out daily tasks such as management of medications and finances.

Alzheimer's is the most commonly occurring cause of dementia, accounting for about 60 to 80 percent of all cases.[30] Although Alzheimer's is not a part of normal aging, it occurs more frequently with increased age, affecting approximately 3 percent of people between ages 65 and 74, 17 percent of people between 75 and 84, and 32 percent of those over 85.[31] In most cases, Alzheimer's begins in the hippocampus, a curled thumb-shaped structure situated about 1.5 inches into the center of brain, behind each ear. The hippocampus functions like a bustling switchboard, rapidly packaging and sending memory-related information to different brain regions for further processing and storage. If plaques and tangles start to gather in the hippocampus, they make it increasingly difficult to process new memories; this is why memory problems are often the first symptom of Alzheimer's. Situated near the left hippocampus (for most right-handed individuals) are brain regions that assist with word knowledge. In Alzheimer's, plaques and tangles often initially form in those regions; this is why increased word-finding difficulties (especially for nouns) is another common early symptom. As the disease progresses, it eventually spreads to other parts of the brain in a fairly predictable pattern. However, clinical symptoms may not begin until 30 years or more after the earliest Alzheimer's-related cellular abnormalities begin to form.[32]

Autopsy studies of people clinically suspected to have Alzheimer's have revealed additional brain abnormalities.[33] The most common include vascular compromise (evidence of small strokes and neuronal damage from insufficient blood supply) and protein abnormalities linked to other types of dementia.[34] The discovery of Alzheimer's-related cellular changes in the presence of other cellular abnormalities has created new opportunities for research that one day may help us find new ways to treat Alzheimer's.

Treatment of Alzheimer's

Prescription memory medication sometimes slows the rate of memory decline in some individuals with Alzheimer's but does not cure the disease or change its underlying cellular pathology. However, recent research has shown that moderate- to high-intensity aerobic exercise can actually change the underlying cellular abnormalities in Alzheimer's.

For example, aerobic exercise can decrease the rate of hippocampal shrinkage.[35] Aerobic exercise also can slow the rate of cognitive decline (as revealed in an analysis of over 800 individuals in 18 randomized controlled trials).[36]

In 2017, a panel of experts reviewed 27 scientific studies and issued a consensus statement on the state of the science regarding exercise and Alzheimer's, finding that:

> Regular participation in physical activity is associated with a reduced risk of developing Alzheimer's disease. Among older adults with Alzheimer's disease and other dementias, regular physical activity can improve performance of activities of daily living and mobility, and may improve general cognition and balance.[37]

Other treatments that can reduce the rate of cognitive decline in individuals with Alzheimer's include cognitive engagement (e.g., discussions of current activities),[38] music therapy,[39] and religion and spirituality[40] (which may relate to social engagement and the development of coping strategies to accept the disease, maintain hope, and find meaning).[41] A clinical trial examining multiple lifestyle treatments is under way (the Multimodal Preventive Trial for Alzheimer's Disease [MIND-AD][42]), and the results are eagerly awaited by the Alzheimer's community.

WHAT IS MILD COGNITIVE IMPAIRMENT?

Mild cognitive impairment (MCI) is a type of accelerated aging that affects about 4.5 percent of people between ages 60 and 69, 5.8 percent of people between 70 and 79, and 7.1 percent of people 80 to 89.[43] MCI is diagnosed when an individual both reports and exhibits cognitive decline compared with a historical "baseline" level, which is also beyond normal age-related decline. However, individuals with MCI generally maintain the ability to manage instrumental activities of daily living (IADLs) (tasks that support independent functioning, such as management of finances, medication, and household needs). In some cases, MCI worsens over time and progresses to dementia (including Alzheimer's or other types of dementia). In other cases, MCI is stable or may even improve. The main criterion that differentiates MCI from dementia is that dementia involves an inability to effectively manage tasks that are necessary for daily functioning.

Treatment of MCI

Randomized controlled trials have shown that aerobic exercise decreases levels of tau[44] (in MCI related to Alzheimer's disease) and reduces shrinkage of the cortex across the entire brain.[45] A major clinical trial, Exercise in Adults with Mild Memory Problems[46] (EXERT), is investigating the impact of physical exercise on brain atrophy, blood flow, cellular markers of Alzheimer's, cognitive ability, and daily functioning in adults with MCI ages 65 to 89.

The Mediterranean diet can slow progression from MCI to Alzheimer's,[47] and mindfulness, yoga, and tai chi are associated with improved memory, attention, and daily functioning.[48] Treatments that involve multiple interventions also show great promise. For example, HABIT (Healthy Action to Benefit Independence & Thinking) is a program that includes memory training, cognitive exercise, yoga, wellness education, and support groups for individuals with MCI and their care partners. HABIT participants report improved daily functioning, mood, and quality of life, among other positive changes (see appendix 2 on pages 231–39 for an interview with Dr. Melanie Chandler, the director of HABIT at the Mayo Clinic in Florida, to learn more about how this pioneering program helps enhance the lives of those with MCI and their partners).

QUIZ: IS IT A BRAIN BLIP OR A MORE CONCERNING MEMORY PROBLEM?

Let's apply what we know about normal and accelerated aging to one of the most common questions people ask about their memory. Circle the item numbers of the following situations that you experience periodically:

1. Forgetting the location of commonly used items such as keys, glasses, a purse, and/or a wallet

2. Forgetting why you walked into a room

3. Forgetting the location of a well-known grocery store

4. Difficulty thinking of the exact word you want to say

5. Forgetting the name of someone you just met

6. Forgetting the name of a close family member or close friend

7. A delay in recalling the name (or forgetting the name) of a casual acquaintance you haven't seen in many years

8. Forgetting an item you intended to buy at the store

9. Forgetting how to do a favorite hobby (e.g., the steps involved in cooking, gardening, or woodworking)

10. Repeatedly forgetting the names of common objects (e.g., "shoes," "car," "dog")

Items 1, 2, 4, 5, 7, and 8 are associated with brain blips and reflect common memory problems that many people experience. Items 3, 6, 9, and 10 are uncommon memory problems, though they can occur for reasons other than an underlying memory disorder (see page 47, Navigational Force 2).

Three Warning Signs of a Potential Memory Problem

1. *Current memory is notably weaker for well-known, frequently used information than before, as evidenced by increasing forgetfulness.* This might include forgetting a well-known recipe or a familiar procedure at work, or forgetting how to navigate to a well-frequented location. Forgetting this sort of familiar information goes beyond brain blips such as failing to find a location you've been to only a couple of times, forgetting to run an errand, and not being able to recall information you never fully learned.

2. *Increased or new forgetfulness that can't be explained.* Increasing forgetfulness for recent events (conversations, activities, and appointments) and/or newfound difficulty managing daily tasks because of memory problems (inability to recall taking medication or paying bills, for example) may be problematic. This is particularly true if the forgetfulness cannot be explained by a known medical, emotional, or situational issue. Some people experience temporary memory problems from stress, lack of sleep, side effects of medication, or medical issues, but memory tends to bounce back after the underlying issue is corrected. Also, it's important to note that forgetting childhood memories and other "remote" information from many years ago is not a common early indicator of a memory problem (though it may occur in the later stages of a memory disorder), and waiting for this type of memory problem to appear could result in a delay in seeking help.

3. *Others have noticed that your memory is worsening.* It is common for people with a memory problem not to be fully aware of it, because they may not remember their own forgetfulness. Often, those we spend the most time with are the first to notice a memory problem and have a sense of how it has worsened over time.

Forgetfulness may be a potential problem if it

- Notably increases from prior levels
- Does not improve when mitigating factors (stress, lack of sleep, medication, etc.) are addressed, and worsens over time
- Involves forgetfulness of well-known information
- Impairs performance of familiar tasks
- Is noticeable to others

If you or a loved one has any or all of these warning signs, it does not mean that there is a definite memory disorder, particularly because memory can be influenced by dozens of factors. Rather, it indicates that you should discuss memory concerns with a health-care provider. This could lead to a workup to investigate possible contributing factors (see page 47, Navigational Force 2).

Now that we have reviewed the trajectories of normal and accelerated aging, let's turn our attention to the last—and strongest—brain health trajectory: the High-Octane Brain.

TRAJECTORY 3: HIGH-OCTANE BRAIN

The top line in figure 1 on page 10 represents the trajectory of optimal aging, or the High-Octane Brain. A High-Octane Brain is one experienced by people with high levels of brain-healthy habits and many of the following outcomes:

- Decreased rate of Alzheimer's
- Reduced rate of age-related brain shrinkage (atrophy)
- Slowed rate of cognitive aging
- Delayed expression of Alzheimer's symptoms
- Decreased rate of Alzheimer's-related cellular abnormalities in the brain
- Enhanced well-being and happiness

Although heredity shapes our brain health trajectory, it doesn't fully define it. Even individuals with a genetic risk for Alzheimer's and those with Alzheimer's-related cellular changes can minimize the impact of these factors on their brain health by integrating brain-healthy habits. Hundreds of studies have shown that culturally diverse individuals with generally average intellectual abilities, with *and* without a hereditary risk for Alzheimer's, have been able to enhance their brain health with specific brain-healthy lifestyle factors and, in some cases, even change the expression of their genetics.

A High-Octane Brain is defined by whether an individual has achieved his or her personal best brain health trajectory by incorporating high levels of brain-healthy habits. The High-Octane Tracker, which you will begin to use in part 2, integrates the top-five brain-healthy habits that will help you achieve a High-Octane Brain.

But how did we come to learn that a High-Octane Brain is even possible? As with many health-related breakthroughs, inspirational role models showed us the way.

The Fabulous Four

Olga Kotelko, who set 37 athletic world records and won 750 track and field medals between the ages of 77 and 95, was an athletic inspiration to people of all ages. What some don't realize is that Olga was also a Brain Health Myth Buster in that she advanced our knowledge of brain health by defying myths about brain aging. At age 93, she had extensive brain imaging and neuropsychological testing that showed that her brain functioned similarly to the brains of women who were decades younger. In particular, the white-matter tracts in her brain—where information is shuttled rapidly between different regions, supporting skills such as reasoning, planning, attention, and information processing—looked especially youthful, particularly in the area that connects the right and left hemispheres of the brain (the corpus callosum). Olga also outperformed her peers on tasks of memory and information processing speed. It was believed that her regular exercise from age 77 on contributed to her exceptional brain health.[49] Olga's story helped overturn the popular myths that brain structure and function are always consistent with chronological age and that exercise started late in life does not improve brain functioning. Her story also debunked the myth that brain functioning in older adults couldn't match that of people decades younger.

Olga's excellent brain health was merely one of her many impressive traits. She also enjoyed a wonderful quality of life, as is often the case for individuals with great brain health. She greeted each day with laughter and was deeply involved with her children and grandchildren, her friends, her faith, and her community. She was also an author and loved Sudoku puzzles. She believed that maintaining an optimistic attitude was the foundation for her many years of excellent health. When she died in 2014, her obituary contained one of her most popular messages, which she wholly embodied: "Don't focus on your age. Focus on how you age."

Although it's not possible to know if Olga's athleticism, positive attitude, and deep involvement in life contributed to her superior brain health, data from multiple studies show that these habits and traits were similar to those of other Brain Health Myth Busters.

The Nun Study is an ongoing research project that has examined the activities, daily functioning, cognitive abilities, and brain autopsies of 678 Roman Catholic nuns from the School Sisters of Notre Dame congregation in Minnesota since 1986. The nuns in the study range in age from 75 to 106. The study has offered often surprising insights about Alzheimer's. In many ways, nuns are an ideal group to study because their brain health is not typically affected by substance use and extensive school and health records allow researchers to learn about their previous experiences and also traits that may have impacted their later brain health. With these sorts of controls, the results of the Nun Study have been integral to our understanding of optimal brain aging.

One of the main findings of the study is that traits and experiences in early, middle, and late life are strongly related to the development of Alzheimer's disease. For example, the linguistic density (complexity of ideas) of autobiographical essays written by the nuns at around age 22 was a significant predictor of developing Alzheimer's. A full 80 percent of nuns whose writing was low in linguistic density went on to develop Alzheimer's, compared with only 10 percent of those who exhibited high linguistic density.[50] Another core finding was that the presence of small strokes increased the risk and severity of Alzheimer's. This finding has been replicated in several studies since then and emphasizes the vital interaction between cardiovascular functioning and Alzheimer's (for more on this, see page 47).

Perhaps most surprisingly, although nuns with greater levels of Alzheimer's-related cellular abnormalities discovered during autopsy had greater memory impairment during life (as expected), the finding did not apply to everyone. *Sister Matthias* was one of the first sisters to participate in the Nun Study and was known as the gold standard for healthy aging. She was vivacious and happily involved in various activities, including knitting mittens for the poor and teaching others how to knit, until her death a few weeks before her 105th birthday.[51] She was another Brain Health Myth Buster. Although her brain had a moderate level of the cellular changes associated with Alzheimer's disease at autopsy—including a spread of the cellular abnormalities to her hippocampus (a core memory area)—she showed no symptoms of Alzheimer's in daily life. Thus, she helped overturn the myth that Alzheimer's-related cellular changes are always expressed in daily life as a problem with memory or other thinking skills.

She wasn't the only one. *Sister Bernadette,* a teacher, had both a genetic risk for Alzheimer's and Alzheimer's-related brain changes at autopsy. However, like Sister Matthias, she never expressed symptoms of Alzheimer's in her daily life. She also had very high performance on tests of memory and other cognitive functioning at ages 81, 83, and 84 before her death at age 85, and she showed no decline on memory testing over time.[52]

Similar case studies emerged to support this exception. *Sister Mary* had eight years of formal education before earning a high school diploma at age 41 and worked as a teacher until she retired at age 84. Even during her retirement, she stayed active in her community, read newspapers and books, prayed for children in different continents on different days of the week, and showed a keen interest in global events. For years before her death just before her 102nd birthday, her performance on cognitive testing remained strong. Similar to Sister Matthias and Sister Bernadette, her brain contained an abundance of cellular abnormalities associated with Alzheimer's, but she never expressed symptoms of the disease.[53]

The Fabulous Four—Olga Kotelko, Sister Matthias, Sister Bernadette, and Sister Mary—challenged established notions about the resilience and functioning of the aging brain even in the context of Alzheimer's-related changes. Similar findings have been noted in individuals from the Rush Memory and Aging Project[54] and in many other studies.

 Individuals with Alzheimer's-related cellular changes in the brain sometimes don't express memory problems or other symptoms of Alzheimer's.

SuperAgers

One important way researchers have learned about healthy brain aging is by studying rare individuals who age *exceptionally*. We refer to these people as SuperAgers. SuperAgers are at least 80 years old and have memory skills on a par with those of 50- to 60-year-olds, if not stronger. Compared with their peers of the same age, they also show less than half the rate of shrinkage in the cortex (the outer layer of the brain, involved in complex information processing). For example, over an 18-month period, while their peers exhibited cortical shrinkage of 2.24 percent, SuperAgers exhibited cortical shrinkage of only 1.06 percent.[55]

Dr. Sandra Weintraub on SuperAgers

Dr. Sandra Weintraub is a professor of psychiatry, behavioral sciences, and neurology at Northwestern University Feinberg School of Medicine. Dr. Weintraub and her colleagues Drs. Marsel Mesulam, Emily Rogalski, and Changiz Geula created the now global concept of SuperAgers. Research on SuperAgers has provided fascinating—and sometimes surprising—insights about this rare group of individuals.

How did you become interested in the concept of SuperAgers?

"All of us . . . we're academic neurologists, neuropsychologists, psychiatrists, social workers . . . and we're also clinicians. . . . We studied dementia so much, and it's really hard to watch people get worse over time. And lots of us knew these anecdotal stories about people who don't go that path, who have a different trajectory. And so we became really interested in the upside of aging, and we decided not to study 'normal aging' but rather to try to handpick people who are functioning at a level well beyond what is considered 'normal' for their age and even 'normal' for a much younger person."

> **"WE'RE HOPING TO JOIN THE RANKS OF SUPERAGERS. WE'RE ALL TRAINING FOR SUPERAGING."**

Dr. Weintraub explained that SuperAgers are classified by their performance on a difficult test of list learning, the Rey Auditory Verbal Learning Test. She noted that some SuperAgers even have total recall of the list after 30 minutes. She explained, "There weren't many other qualifications beyond extraordinary memory, other than you couldn't have a prior diagnosis of a psychiatric or neurological disorder. Although some of our participants had a stroke midstudy, they couldn't have it going in. We just thought, 'Really, this is interesting. Let's study this trajectory and try to figure it out. Can we learn something from it that we can then write a prescription for how to do this?'"

What has been most surprising about your work with SuperAgers?

"Our center has a theme. We call it 'heterogeneity [variability] of cognitive aging and dementia.' What's so striking to us is how different older people are from one another. As people age, they take very different pathways, and I think the most important thing is to try to understand those that are in that upper echelon. But there's no prescription for it." Dr. Weintraub discussed several surprising findings in SuperAgers, including the following:

Some SuperAgers have significant life stress. She noted, "So you would think that severe stress during your life would damage your hippocampus. We have Holocaust survivors. I don't think you can get any higher on the stress scale than that."

Some SuperAgers have cellular evidence of Alzheimer's. "There are some SuperAgers that have one silly neurofibrillary tangle in the hippocampus. One." She noted that conversely, other SuperAgers had evidence of Alzheimer's neuropathologic change on postmortem brain autopsy but did not express related symptoms.

SuperAger educational levels are variable. "We have people with very high levels of education. Then we have people with a high school education or less than high school."

Are there commonalities among SuperAgers?

Although variability among SuperAgers is notable, Dr. Weintraub explained, some commonalities have emerged:

Resilience: "Neuroticism [being prone to experiencing negative emotions] is very low in this sample, and despite what's happened to them in life, they're amazingly resilient. There's part of it that's biology and then part of it that's lifestyle. They have psychological resilience, and they have neuropathologic resilience." Dr. Weintraub described how difficult it is to measure resilience, noting, "I think that we don't really know how to measure resilience. We can give questionnaires. We can look at neurons . . . what we're trying to understand is what is this resilience they have."

Social engagement: Dr. Weintraub noted that although not all SuperAgers are extroverts, "These people, as a group, are highly social. They like to be with people. They are very interactive. They have social networks. We've had a couple of SuperAger parties because they have insisted that we have parties for them. These are parties where they want music and they want to dance. They're very engaged. They just want to connect."

Dr. Weintraub discussed the idea that von Economo neurons, which process social information, may represent a potential biological underpinning of SuperAger social engagement and that such neurons "are only found in social animals, which is kind of the initial hypothesis we had and why we specifically looked at those neurons." She noted that SuperAgers have four to five times greater density in von Economo neurons than their cognitively normal-for-age controls.

SuperAger resilience and social engagement are long-standing traits, Dr. Weintraub explained. "This is nothing new. It's not something they've developed in older age," she added. Dr. Weintraub and her team are also looking at SuperAger life stories to better understand other characteristics of this rare group that are not easily quantified.

Can others cultivate the traits of SuperAgers?

Dr. Weintraub noted that although there is no prescription for SuperAging, "I think there's a lesson to be learned. Knowing what your weaknesses are is really important. So if you're in your thirties, forties, or fifties and you are neurotic [prone to experiencing negative emotions], get treated. Our mantra is 'Treat what you can'—sleep disorders, depression, alcohol abuse, exercise, diet. Do whatever you can do that's not going to hurt you. That's our prescription. And it's not going to cost to pay for online training that is not proven."

Dr. Weintraub added, "I think that there's a combination of nature and nurture, so that we cannot ignore either one or the other. . . . People need to be aware of what are their risks, so if they have [genetic problems], they're going to have to go way overboard on the nurture side. And if they have good genetics . . . they probably could even do better if they keep the nurture up with the level of the genetics. So I think it's kind of a combination of those factors, and people just need to be aware."

SuperAger Overview

1. *Our early life experiences are just some of the many factors that drive our brain health trajectories.* Many SuperAgers had early life experiences that would seem likely to compromise their future brain health, including significant stress and low levels of education.

2. *Emotional resilience, social engagement, and lower amounts of negative emotions are common and lifelong among SuperAgers.* Social engagement may relate to a greater number of von Economo neurons, but overall these findings provide support for the potential role of positive emotional factors in brain health (more on this in chapter 7).

3. *Nature and nurture are vital to determining brain health.* Knowing your family history, your strengths, and your weaknesses can help you determine what actions to take to maximize your brain health. The intersection of these issues will be explored throughout this book.

OPTIMAL BRAIN AGING

Optimal brain aging can be defined in a "norm-referenced" way in which an individual's functioning is judged to be superior to that of his or her peers. This is the case with SuperAgers, who score significantly higher on memory testing than their same-age peers based on normative data. Optimal brain aging also can be defined as "criterion-referenced," in which individuals are assessed according to the level at which they meet specific criteria, such as how much they integrate brain-healthy habits.[56] The High-Octane Brain is based on a criterion-referenced definition that measures the level at which an individual incorporates the brain-healthy habits linked to a decreased rate of memory decline and brain shrinkage, a decreased risk of Alzheimer's, and enhanced well-being. When a criterion-referenced approach is used to define optimal aging, a High-Octane Brain becomes a possible outcome for almost every individual. That's great news because we can't all be SuperAgers!

TOP TAKEAWAYS

By 2050, the global population of older adults will double and the global rate of Alzheimer's will triple. The following game-changing rules of brain aging provide powerful guidance to decrease the rate of Alzheimer's and boost brain health:

1. Although there are genetic risk factors associated with Alzheimer's (much more on that in chapter 2), there is no direct genetic cause for 99 percent of cases of Alzheimer's. Although lifestyle factors are not the only factor involved in the disease, they are the most powerful proven tool we have to decrease the rate of Alzheimer's and delay its onset.

2. For many people, Alzheimer's is "silent" for decades, and symptoms may not start for 30 years or more after related cellular changes have occurred. The best defense against Alzheimer's is a proactively healthy lifestyle, especially since there is no cure for the disease.

3. Brain Health Myth Busters show that it's not inevitable to express symptoms of Alzheimer's even if Alzheimer's-related brain changes are present.

4. Our brain health trajectory—whether in line with the path of normal aging, accelerated aging, or the High-Octane Brain—is determined by far more than our genetics and early life experiences. Our behavior and habits are pivotal. The High-Octane Brain is associated with a significantly decreased risk of Alzheimer's, a decreased rate of age-related brain shrinkage, and a slowed rate of cognitive aging.

5. SuperAgers are providing insights that will help us learn more about optimal brain aging. Research is under way to learn more about this incredible (and rare) group of individuals.

6. The lifestyle habits associated with the High-Octane Brain are not only our best defense against Alzheimer's, they're also the best tools we have to enhance our overall brain health and all that extends from it, including improved well-being and overall health.

CHAPTER 2

The Journey Begins

"Goals transform a random walk into a chase."

—Mihaly Csikszentmihalyi

"Please help me improve my memory. I'll do anything to avoid Alzheimer's," Meredith said, leaning forward in her chair, looking at me intently.

I'd seen the same look from Meredith, age 58, when she'd arrived late for the introductory meeting of my seven-week High-Octane Brain class the week prior. The class met weekly to focus on a different aspect of brain health and to discuss how to create a personalized High-Octane Brain Action Plan and follow the weekly brain health tracking system, the High-Octane Tracker (see appendix 1 on pages 214–30). Although all the class members shared a desire to enhance their memory and reduce their risk of Alzheimer's, a few had already started to notice concerning memory changes.

Before the introductory meeting, the members were provided with guidance to ensure that the class was a fit for them. They learned that people without an existing memory diagnosis such as Alzheimer's or MCI probably would get the strongest benefit from the program. However, they also learned that multiple High-Octane Brain strategies are therapeutic for individuals with Alzheimer's and MCI.

PREPARING FOR YOUR JOURNEY

Before starting the class, the participants met with their medical providers to discuss their memory concerns and weigh the need for a workup to measure their levels of vitamins, thyroid function, and other issues that can contribute to memory problems. During the introductory meeting, several members said that their medical providers had mentioned the need to better manage their vascular health (diabetes, high blood pressure, and high cholesterol). A few mentioned that they also had been encouraged to stop smoking and lose weight. We discussed how managing these factors can be helpful because they are all significantly linked to memory skills and Alzheimer's. Two members also explained how they'd been referred for a neuropsychological assessment to get a statistical measure of their cognitive functioning (the "software" of the brain). Those who'd gone through this process felt that it helped them better understand and harness their cognitive strengths. They also felt reassured that they now had a precise baseline of their cognitive functioning to help them track changes over time. The members also reviewed the diet and exercise recommendations in the High-Octane Brain plan with their medical providers to ensure that they didn't have any restrictions.

Some members chose to work with another class member as an "accountability partner" to discuss assignments and progress and provide mutual encouragement. You too may choose to work with an accountability partner as you complete the High-Octane Brain program, or you can do the program on your own. If you're not sure which is better for you, think back to how you've successfully made changes in the past. If having a partner or social support enhanced your progress, consider inviting someone to do the program with you. Whether or not you have an accountability partner, you may find it helpful to mention the program and the goal of better brain health to your family and friends. This often provides increased support and encouragement and helps maximize progress.

Everyone in the class expressed a desire to both maximize his or her future memory skills and reduce the risk of Alzheimer's. The discussion got animated quickly after we reviewed research indicating that symptoms of Alzheimer's may not show up until 30 years or more after related cellular changes occur and that even a distant family history of Alzheimer's can increase the risk of developing the disease. Some members were concerned that they had multiple relatives with memory problems, and others—such as Meredith (featured below)—suspected that a relative might have had undiagnosed Alzheimer's. They were reassured that the science behind the High-Octane Brain plan has been shown to be effective for people who do and don't have a genetic risk of Alzheimer's and/or a family history of Alzheimer's or suspected Alzheimer's.

THE FINGER STUDY

A recent research project called the FINGER study (the Finnish Geriatric Intervention Study to Prevent Cognitive Impairment and Disability), a randomized controlled trial on brain health, revealed some very promising results. The study showed that people who followed a healthy lifestyle that included exercise, a brain-healthy diet, cognitive training, and vascular risk management—things such as improving blood pressure and cholesterol—had a 30 percent reduction in cognitive decline after just two years.[57] Those benefits continued for two more years after the study[58] and are still being tracked.

A randomized control trial such as the FINGER study is the gold standard for testing scientific ideas because it allows us to examine cause and effect. In other words, it gives us greater confidence to say that the decreased cognitive decline found in the FINGER study was directly caused by a healthier lifestyle; it wasn't that people had better brain functioning because they were just healthier overall.

Even more exciting, the FINGER study showed that people who were APOE-e4 positive (see pages 45–46)—those with a genetic risk for Alzheimer's—had the *same* level of reduced cognitive decline as those who did not have a genetic risk for Alzheimer's.[59] It is also worth noting that FINGER seemed to be even *more* therapeutic for people with other cognitive impairment risk factors, such as having a less healthy lifestyle and shorter telomeres[60] (the tips of DNA strands). Telomeres get worn and shredded as we age, kind of like the way the caps on the tips of a shoelace get worn over time. They're also a measure of the body's overall cellular aging.

This is where the idea of the High-Octane Brain really matters. No matter what our heredity is, we can enhance the trajectory of our future brain health by integrating specific brain-healthy habits. Although this may not fully prevent Alzheimer's, *a lot* of research suggests that brain-healthy habits can buy time by delaying when Alzheimer's symptoms start, sometimes by more than 10 years.[61]

EPIGENETICS AND THE HIGH-OCTANE BRAIN

Another study that reinforces this idea was done with people who have a rare form of genetically caused Alzheimer's called autosomal-dominant Alzheimer's, which affects only 1 percent of people with the disease. Those with this rare genetic profile are guaranteed to develop Alzheimer's, because they have one of three genes. However, *when* they express symptoms has been shown to vary depending on their lifestyle factors. Those who exercised at high levels were able to delay the diagnosis of Alzheimer's by *15 years* and had stronger cognitive functioning compared with people who exercised at a low level.[62] Amazingly, high exercisers also had significantly lower levels of cellular changes (beta-amyloid plaques) associated with Alzheimer's.[63] In other words, even in a rare genetically caused subtype of Alzheimer's, lifestyle factors were linked to significant differences in brain structure and function.

These sorts of outcomes may be a result of our ability to alter the expression of our genes through our behavior, a branch of science called *epigenetics*. Because we all have different inborn abilities, genetics, and early experiences, each person's highest possible level of brain health will be different. Thus, it's helpful to imagine a High-Octane Brain as the highest level of brain health each of us is capable of: our *personal best*. That level is affected by our "foundational factors," the inborn traits and past events that often influence our brain health trajectory. Foundational factors include our genetics, personality, intellectual capacity, and early life experiences, among other variables (see pages 45–47). However, our behavior can significantly alter the impact of our foundational factors and thus our ultimate brain health trajectory.

For example, some people have a high level of inborn intelligence (a foundational factor) but don't have a healthy lifestyle or don't seek out new learning experiences. They may even have a strong memory and never get Alzheimer's, but they won't develop a High-Octane Brain if they don't integrate the healthy lifestyle factors that allow them to attain their personal best level of brain functioning. Conversely, a person with a lower level of inborn intelligence may attain his or her personal best level of brain functioning by having a healthy lifestyle and seeking out new learning experiences.

This is why we define a High-Octane Brain in terms of reaching our individual maximum brain health capacity, which is based on our adherence to a brain-healthy lifestyle. This is where the High-Octane Tracker comes in; you can use it to measure your adoption of brain-healthy habits at different levels: good, better, and best. The process of changing brain health habits is full of trial and error, and we'll never do it perfectly. However, when we can improve some of our brain health habits, we're making progress.

At the end of the day, pursuing a High-Octane Brain allows us to answer yes to the question "Did I do my best to optimize my brain health and reach my full brain health potential?"

MEREDITH MEETS LOU

To help us better understand the challenges and rewards of following a High-Octane Brain approach to brain health, two members of my seven-week class on the subject—Meredith and Lou—agreed to share their journey toward better brain health. Their progress will be discussed here and in the pages that follow.

At our first meeting, I had a few minutes to chat with Meredith while she waited to meet her accountability partner, Lou, who was running late.

"I'm concerned," she said. "I've been forgetting why I walk into a room, and the other day I couldn't remember my password for a few minutes. I've seen so many people suffer from Alzheimer's, and I want to avoid it at all costs."

Meredith worked as an accountant at the same firm for 30 years and developed close relationships with many long-term clients. She has two children who went on to have four grandchildren, ages 4 to 10. To spend more time with them, she cut back her work schedule from full time to part time six years earlier.

"My kids work full-time, so I've been helping with my grandkids, and I just love it," Meredith explained. "I wasn't able to spend much time with my kids when they were growing up because I was so busy with my career. But I want to be there for my grandkids. They count on me, and I like that."

Her brown eyes were warm and playful when she discussed her life, but her expression shifted quickly as she spoke of her concerns about memory, and her voice trembled: "I'm the youngest of three. My mom had a lot of memory problems. We used to think it was because she was getting older, but when she died at 89, the doctors told us her memory problems weren't normal aging. She wasn't even able to remember my name half the time."

"I was worried she would forget who I was," Meredith continued. "She was never diagnosed with Alzheimer's, but I think she had it." Her voice became softer as she lifted her head and looked me squarely in the eye. "I'll do anything to avoid that and save my family the burden of having to take care of me."

Meredith spoke faster and more quietly. She mentioned family friends who'd been diagnosed with Alzheimer's. Eventually she started to cry: "My clients count on me, and I need to stay sharp for them. I want to do whatever I can to make sure I don't get Alzheimer's. I don't think my family could handle it, and neither could I."

Just then, Lou, a burly man with thinning gray hair and a booming voice, ambled into the room with a tall younger man at his side. "This is my boy, Al," Lou said proudly. Al nodded and quietly sat down next to Lou, across from Meredith.

"I'm sorry, I didn't realize we were supposed to bring someone with us," Meredith said.

"I just came to help him get started with this process." Al said.

"He knows I might not come otherwise," Lou interrupted before a serious look came across his face.

Lou quickly expressed his concerns: "I used to have a great memory, but I'm slipping. It's darn frustrating."

Lou's son looked worried. "He's been about 30 pounds overweight for a long time. It never seemed to impact him much, but now he's slowing down. He's always short of breath and doesn't have much stamina. He used to know all sorts of random facts about cars and baseball. He was like an encyclopedia, but now he's just . . . slower. He talks slower, walks slower . . . he thinks slower. It's been like this for two years, since . . ." His voice trailed off. "And it seems to be getting worse."

Lou looked down after Al spoke. He was quiet for a long time. "I hate it, but he's right," Lou admitted. "But I've always felt healthy, even with my high blood pressure and diabetes."

Meredith sat back in her chair.

Lou was a retired machinist who had been widowed two years earlier. He cried softly when discussing his wife's death.

"I worry about him," Al said. He spends so much time by himself. I'm not sure what he does all day."

Al explained that Lou stopped working on his cars, a lifelong passion. He also shared examples of Lou's disengagement from his usual activities and expressed concern that Lou "didn't seem like his old self." Meredith said she also felt disengaged from what she truly loved to do, but for different reasons. She felt her tendency to prioritize caring for her clients and family left her with "little time for me." Although she'd been fine with that in her earlier years, as she got older and became more concerned about her memory, she realized that she didn't have the time to research brain-healthy habits, much less follow a brain-healthy lifestyle.

For Lou, his disengagement since his wife's death probably would make it challenging to start new brain health habits, but he was willing to try to make positive changes because he had promised his son he would. Meredith realized that the time she spent taking care of others probably would drain her available time to try out new brain health habits. In recognizing these big-picture factors, newcomers to the High-Octane Brain approach can help accelerate the change process and address barriers to progress.

It was an encouraging sign that Meredith and Lou were excited to learn that a High-Octane Brain is linked not only to reduced memory decline and a decreased rate of Alzheimer's but also to higher levels of happiness and well-being. They agreed to meet later that week to share their answers to the first exercises.

How to Use Your High-Octane
Action Plan and High-Octane Tracker

Let's get started on your High-Octane Brain journey, the core of which is the High-Octane Action Plan described on pages 214–15. The Action Plan allows you to personalize your motivation for brain health by completing exercises in each of the chapters.

Whenever you see this thought bubble icon and the word "Reflect," you will be prompted to complete an exercise in the High-Octane Action Plan.

The section after the Action Plan is the High-Octane Tracker (see pages 219–30), which allows you to track the five steps toward better brain health. You will see this arrow icon and the word "Track" whenever you are prompted to complete a portion of the High-Octane Tracker.

Although Meredith and Lou and the rest of the High-Octane Brain class members initially progressed through the program a week at a time, feel free to spend up to two weeks working on each step if you would prefer a slower pace. By continuing to move to the next step every one to two weeks, progress on previous steps is often unexpectedly boosted. This is probably because—as you'll learn—the behaviors start to synergize and create an experience in which the whole is greater than the sum of its parts. For example, improving sleep (the last step in the program) often leads to increased exercise (step 1) and engagement (step 3) and so forth.

Since you will be frequently flipping back to your High-Octane Action Plan and Tracker, it may be helpful to put a bookmark or sticky note on pages 214 and 219, where the Action Plan and Tracker begin, respectively.

HIGH-OCTANE BRAIN ACTION PLAN: YOUR IDEAL FUTURE SELF

A greater sense of purpose in life is associated with a reduced risk of Alzheimer's.[64] This exercise, and the ones that follow throughout the book, encourage you not only to hone your purpose but also to envision what is possible for you and those you love if you pursue a High-Octane Brain. We'll learn about Meredith and Lou's answers to this exercise in chapter 3. In the meantime, let's kick off your Action Plan by putting your Ideal Future Self at the heart of your brain health journey.

 Reflect: Your *Whys*

I encourage you to explore this simple but important question that lies at the heart of this journey:

Why do you want better brain health?

Here are some popular reasons that people cite for why they want better brain health. Do any apply to you?

1. "I want to stay engaged at my highest level in my most important relationships with family members, friends, and colleagues for as long as possible."

2. "I have a family history of memory problems, and I want to reduce my risk of Alzheimer's."

3. "I've started to notice subtle memory changes, and I want to proactively enhance my future memory."

4. "I want to be at the top of my game as I continue my life's work."

5. "I need to be around to take care of my loved ones, and I want to be able to do that as long and effectively as possible."

6. "I know that my ability to manage my health, do my favorite activities, and live independently depends on having the strongest brain health possible."

Do any of these resonate with you? Take a moment to identify your unique "Whys," and write the top two in the "Whys for Better Brain Health" section under the "Chapter 2" heading of your High-Octane Action Plan.

Reflect: Envision Your Ideal Future Self

Step 1: Close your eyes and imagine what you'd be doing if you accomplished the two Whys you just identified. For example, if you chose reason 1 above ("I want to stay engaged at my highest level in my most important relationships with family members, friends, and colleagues for as long as possible"), imagine yourself in a situation in which that occurs.

Step 2: Now imagine yourself accomplishing both of your Whys for better brain health while simultaneously looking as healthy and vibrant as possible. Make the experience multisensory. See, hear, and feel the sensations that accompany this vision. Visualize the elements in detail. For example: Are you by yourself or with others? How do you look? Where are you? Try to conjure as many details as you can. How do you feel? Joyful? Calm? Notice any sensations on your skin. A breeze? The feel of soft fabric?

On your High-Octane Action Plan, in the section titled "Your Ideal Future Self" under the "Chapter 2" heading, jot down three of the most salient details you envisioned. Make sure they are powerful enough to allow you to reimagine this vision easily.

Revisit Your Ideal Future Self

This next part might sound funny, but it's actually a very effective technique to increase motivation for brain health. Think of your Ideal Future Self for about five seconds the next time you brush your teeth. See if you can bring it to mind consistently every time you brush. When you connect it with a daily activity, the vision should stay more top of mind for you and become a stronger motivator. You may notice that your vision starts to develop different details over time as you learn more High-Octane Brain steps.

TOP TAKEAWAYS

1. If you have concerning memory problems, discuss them with a healthcare provider to see if you would benefit from a workup to investigate possible causes of memory change.

2. If you feel social support would boost your progress in developing a High-Octane Brain, consider finding an accountability partner to join you in completing the program.

3. In addition to reducing the risk of Alzheimer's, a High-Octane Brain can buy time by significantly delaying the start of Alzheimer's for people who would otherwise express symptoms much sooner.

4. The FINGER study and other research show the incredible power of behavior in shaping our brain health trajectory whether or not we have a genetic risk for Alzheimer's.

5. High levels of brain-healthy behaviors allow you to attain a High-Octane Brain, your personal best level of brain health, as measured by the High-Octane Tracker (see pages 219–30).

6. Along with Meredith and Lou, you began to personalize your High-Octane Action Plan by visualizing your Ideal Future Self and identifying your *Whys* for better brain health.

CHAPTER 3

A Fresh Start: How to Maximize Your Brain Health

"We are what we repeatedly do. Excellence, then, is not an act but a habit."

—WILL DURANT, SUMMARIZING ARISTOTLE'S INSIGHTS

The promise and majesty of a space shuttle launch is a marvel to behold. The tiniest shifts in its angle of departure are magnified exponentially with every mile it soars as its intricate navigational systems continually nudge it almost imperceptibly toward its destination. It's a powerful example of how trajectory-making is a process, not a single act.

The journey of the High-Octane Brain is similar. It, too, is a journey of promise, one that requires a successful launch and continued adjustments to stay the course. The difference between space and health journeys, though, is that in a health journey the benefits we expect upon reaching our destination are present almost immediately, as soon as we begin to incorporate brain-healthy behaviors. For example, growing research shows the immediate benefits of exercise, sleep, and stress management on memory functioning, and those benefits aggregate over time, providing stronger memory and a reduced risk of Alzheimer's. In other words, the fruits of the journey are present right away *and* in the future. The journey itself is powered by the realization that at any given moment our choices put us on the trajectory of our making, regardless of how our foundational factors—the inborn traits and past events that often influence our brain health trajectory (see page 33)—have launched us.

Dr. Marwan Sabbagh on Changing Your Mind-Set

Dr. Marwan Sabbagh is a board-certified neurologist, director of the Cleveland Clinic Lou Ruvo Center for Brain Health, and clinical professor in the Department of Neurology at the University of Nevada, Las Vegas.

What are the most helpful brain health interventions?

"The reality is we have to engage in wellness and brain health in all aspects: diet, exercise, stress management, sleeping, and managing and optimizing your health conditions. Everything. It's not one thing. It's not like you can live a terrible life and eat a terrible diet and then buy a whole row of supplements and say that's good enough. It just doesn't work that way. You have to do it all."

Dr. Sabbagh discussed exercise as one of the most beneficial strategies to begin with when one is adopting a brain-healthy lifestyle. "I think that's one of the quickest things," he added.

Can you describe why the concept of epigenetics (the ability to change the expression of our genes through our behavior) is so powerful?

"There are many things in our life—whether it's diet, exercise, stress, or sleep—that can turn on or turn off genes through something called DNA methylation. We think, of course, that diet is one of the most impactful and immediate ways to alter your epigenetics."

Dr. Sabbagh believes that it's important for people to experience a "mind-set change" when it comes to the power of lifestyle interventions. "The fundamental issue is that people are skeptical," he said. "They believe the only solutions are going to come out of an infusion or a pill. They can't believe that something like a lifestyle intervention would make the difference."

However, he explained, it's difficult to tease apart the roles of genetics and lifestyle factors in people who age optimally, noting, "I don't think we have explained their genetic propensity to safeguard their brain . . . the fundamental issue being that those people who do those things are generally healthy to begin with."

Are supplements helpful in maximizing brain health?

"Supplements are controversial. The World Health Organization and the National Academy of Sciences looked very carefully at supplements, and both groups came to the same conclusion that there was insufficient data to support the recommendation of supplements for brain health. Despite that, they're very popular and very highly consumed and very, very heavily marketed whether there's good data or not.

"Supplements, in fact, have to meet a standard called GRAS, or Generally Recognized as Safe. They have to show they're as safe as a potato chip. They do not have to show any measure of efficacy . . . it's basically largely unregulated as an industry. So what you see is that a lot of things get promoted and recommended when there's not a shred of evidence to support it."

What are the best ways to put brain-healthy habits into action?

"I often lecture about the point that change is hard. If you are a sedentary person and your doctor is wagging his finger at you and saying 'Okay, you need to exercise now,' no matter how well intended you are, it doesn't happen easily. . . . Start slowly and incrementally. It's the long view. You're not saying 'Go out and run a marathon tomorrow.' Say 'Okay, start on a specific low-impact regimen and grow it from there, and get your body used to a change.'"

> "PEOPLE UNFORTUNATELY WAIT UNTIL SOME CATASTROPHIC EVENT OCCURS BEFORE THEY DECIDE TO DO SOMETHING THAT WOULD ALTER THEIR RISK."

How do you build brain health into your own busy life?

"First of all, I built my life and schedule around it. I try to exercise every morning when I wake up. And I built my schedule around getting up at a specific time, walking the dog, going to exercise. And that's how I start my day every morning. I really get upset and annoyed when something happens in my schedule that prevents, delays, and does not allow me to have my schedule. So harmony in my schedule is very important."

"It's difficult if it's competing against something else," he added. "Time is everybody's enemy. It's all about competing priorities. I was still trying to do these things when my kids were at home and not in college yet, so I just made it a priority."

Dr. Sabbagh noted that like most people, he is working to increase his use of some brain health techniques. "I work very hard to sleep well. The first time I ever meditated in my life—I'm 53 years old—was in 2019, so that's something I started to do. . . . I wish I'd do more, but change is hard."

"You've got to build your life around these things, right? So diet . . . is a conscious thing. When you open the refrigerator, you can either eat a doughnut or eat egg whites or eat something else. The bottom line is you're going to put food in your mouth. It's just a matter of choosing what you're putting in your mouth. So part of it is a schedule, and part of it is a deliberate, intentional, mindful choice."

THE POWER OF EPIGENETICS

As Dr. Sabbagh mentioned, there is increasing evidence that we can alter the ways in which our genes are expressed—sometimes even turning them on or off—through our behavior.

It's as if our genetics and our behavior are dance partners that both have the power to lead and to modify the direction of the dance. That realization puts us on a different playing field from the popular assumption that the expression of our genetics cannot be altered. When we see that gene expression is a dance and not a predestined process, it provides hope and excitement about our ability to shift our brain health trajectory. It underlines that we truly are in control of our brain and can change its future. It also sets the stage for an exploration of the three Navigational Forces that form our individual brain health trajectory.

 The science of epigenetics shows that we can alter the ways our genes are expressed—sometimes even turning them on or off—through our behavior.

The Three Navigational Forces

Each of the three brain health trajectories that we learned about in chapter 1—normal aging, accelerated aging, and optimal aging/High-Octane Brain—results from the combined effects of three navigational forces. (The first two navigational forces are altered by the third navigational force, which is lifestyle factors.)

Navigational Force 1: Foundational Factors

Our foundational factors—our genetics, historical factors, and age—strongly influence our brain health trajectory. But these factors were generally established in the past; some are associated with an increased risk of Alzheimer's, whereas others can lead to a decreased risk. Although epigenetics can modify the way some of these core factors are expressed, they may still affect our brain health trajectory. Here's a breakdown:

- **Age.** Age is the greatest risk factor for cognitive impairment, including Alzheimer's.

- **Genetics.** There is no direct genetic cause for 99 percent of cases of Alzheimer's. However, the APOE gene on chromosome 19, which is related to cholesterol transport in the blood, has been linked to an increased risk, a decreased risk, or a neutral risk of Alzheimer's. Like many genes, the APOE gene has two *alleles*, or genetic sequences: one inherited from each parent. The e2 ("E two" or "epsilon two") allele is linked to a reduced risk of Alzheimer's (present in about 5 percent of the population); the e3 allele is linked to a neutral risk of Alzheimer's (present in about 75 percent of the population); and the e4 allele is linked to a higher risk of Alzheimer's (present in about 20 percent of the population).[65] Having one copy of the e4 allele increases the risk of developing Alzheimer's 2 to 5 times, and having two copies increases the risk 9 to 12 times. However, since many individuals with the *APOE*-e4 gene live into their nineties and approximately 75 percent of individuals with Alzheimer's have no family history of Alzheimer's disease,[66] there are clearly nongenetic factors involved in the development of Alzheimer's.

- **Family history of Alzheimer's.** A 2019 study showed that people with one first-degree relative (a parent, sibling, or child) with Alzheimer's had almost twice the risk of developing the disease.[67] Having two first-degree relatives was linked to a nearly 4 times higher risk of developing the disease, and having four first-degree relatives was linked to a 15 times higher risk. People with three or four second-degree relatives (grandparents, grandchildren, aunts, uncles, nieces, and nephews) with Alzheimer's were more than twice as likely to develop the disease. People with the lowest risk had no relatives with the disease or only one or two third-degree relatives with the disease.[68]

- **Educational level.** Individuals with higher levels of education have a lower risk of Alzheimer's; this may relate to higher levels of cognitive reserve (see chapter 6, page 113).

- **Lifelong bilingualism.** This is associated with a delayed expression of dementia by approximately 4 to 5 years.[69]

Note that biological sex and ethnicity are also foundational factors. Although the expression of these factors is not typically modified in the realm of brain health, it is important to note that they can affect our brain health trajectory. For example:

- **Women** are twice as likely as men to be diagnosed with Alzheimer's. Although much is still unknown about sex differences and the risk of Alzheimer's, some research suggests that women may have greater vulnerability to developing the disease, possibly related to hormonal factors.[70]

- **Ethnicity.** Compared with white Americans, African Americans are more than twice as likely to develop Alzheimer's and Hispanic Americans are more than 1.5 times as likely.[71] Worldwide, regional estimates of Alzheimer's through 2050 range from 4.7 percent in Central Europe to 8.7 percent in Northern Africa, with all other world regions ranging between 5.6 and 7.6 percent.[72]

Navigational Force 2: Health-Related Factors

The expression "What is good for the heart is good for the brain" captures the essence of much research on the relationship between cardiovascular health and Alzheimer's. There is strong evidence that vascular risk factors such as high blood pressure, high cholesterol, and diabetes are strongly linked to higher than average brain shrinkage and cognitive decline[73] and an increased risk of Alzheimer's. The data is mixed on whether a previous history of head injury increases the future likelihood of Alzheimer's.[74] However, epilepsy (seizures), sleep apnea, obesity, smoking, excessive alcohol use, and anticholinergic medications (which block the action of the neurotransmitter acetylcholine, which is crucial to memory) are linked to an increased risk of memory problems and/or Alzheimer's. Having one or more of these issues is not cause for panic. In conjunction with a medical provider, many people are able to improve several health-related factors, such as smoking, alcohol use, high blood pressure, high cholesterol, diabetes, and even sleep apnea.

Navigational Force 3: Lifestyle Factors

The five science-backed lifestyle factors that you will learn about in part 2 have the power to maximally upgrade the brain health trajectory impacted by Navigational Forces 1 and 2. In fact, their influence is so significant that they function as the *inflection point*: the point at which the direction of a person's brain health trajectory has the maximum ability to be modified. These factors influence our brain health trajectory in the following ways:

A. Through positive cellular changes, including increased growth hormones, circulation, and oxygenation, and through increased removal of toxic proteins.

B. By modifying Navigational Force 1 (foundational factors), including genetics, historical events, and age—through epigenetics and the behaviors that affect the expression of other historical factors (compensating for any negative impact of childhood experiences, limited educational opportunities, previous injuries, etc.).

C. By modifying Navigational Force 2 (health-related factors). For example, a brain-healthy lifestyle often has a positive impact on other areas of health and can result in improvement of blood pressure, cholesterol, diabetes, obesity, smoking, and excessive alcohol use.

Positive lifestyle factors create a synergistic positive feedback loop that increases our ability to continue living a brain-healthy lifestyle. The stronger our brain functioning is, the better able we are to plan, implement, evaluate, and revise our lifestyle choices.[75] For example, when we exercise, we are more likely to sleep well (among several other areas of improvement), and by sleeping well, we are more likely to have the energy to exercise. Improved exercise and sleep are in turn associated with many other positive effects, including enhanced memory, well-being, and health. In addition, higher levels of omega-3 fatty acids have been shown to reduce the negative impact of low levels of exercise,[76] and a healthy diet minimizes recurrent depression.[77] The series of positive feedback loops we experience from enhanced brain health gain momentum over time and can become a powerful self-sustaining tool to bolster our brain health trajectory.

THE EXCELS METHOD

The High-Octane Brain Tracker incorporates five lifestyle factors that have been shown to have the strongest ability to shift our brain health trajectory, especially when used in combination. The acronym EXCELS helps us remember the lifestyle factors and the order in which they are used in the tracking system:

Step 1: **EX**ercise is the X-Factor

Step 2: **C**onsume Healthy Food

Step 3: **E**ngage and Learn!

Step 4: **L**ower Stress and Boost Well-Being

Step 5: **S**leep for Brain Power

When maintained consistently and integrated at high levels, these steps are the path to a High-Octane Brain. They gain added power when used in conjunction with improvements in any personal risk factors you may have (Navigational Forces 1 and 2).

The five steps in the EXCELS Method were selected on the basis of the following considerations:

1. *A review of the literature on factors that maximize brain health and also minimize the risk of Alzheimer's.* The order of the steps is based on the strength and size of the data showing that a particular step significantly alters the trajectory of brain health and decreases the risk of Alzheimer's. It's possible that some lifestyle factors have stronger support simply because they have been studied longer and more deeply, and the ordering of the steps doesn't imply that later steps are not as important as earlier steps. For example, although sleep could easily be viewed as the most important step (because good sleep is necessary to carry out all the other steps), it's listed as the last step because the research on improving sleep to decrease the risk of Alzheimer's is not as strong

as the research on the power of exercise and diet (steps 1 and 2) to do the same thing. Also, because the first three EXCELS steps have comparatively more research support for enhancing brain health, you'll notice that they can be tracked with more precision than can the latter two steps in the High-Octane Tracker.

2. *The 2019 World Health Organization (WHO) Guidelines for Risk Reduction of Cognitive Decline and Dementia.*[78] These guidelines provide support for integrating exercise, a brain-healthy diet, and cognitive engagement into a brain health plan. Although stress management and sleep are not recommended in the WHO Guidelines, they're included in the EXCELS Method because emerging research suggests that they provide powerful opportunities to enhance brain health and decrease the risk of Alzheimer's.[79] All the WHO recommendations have been incorporated into the High-Octane Brain plan either through the EXCELS Method or through coverage of individual risk factors (Navigational Forces 1 and 2).

3. *A recognition that multiple factors maximize brain health, as discussed by Dr. Sabbagh* (see pages 42–44).

The EXCELS Method includes five science-backed steps that have shown the greatest effectiveness in enhancing brain health and decreasing the risk of Alzheimer's.

MAKING A CHOICE

We are at the center of our trajectory making. We have the power at any given moment to choose a brain-healthy behavior. Every behavior—whether it's what we will eat, in what activity we will engage, how much we will sleep, or how we will cope with stress—involves a Three-Path Choice (see figure 2). At some point, every decision you make involves answering yes to one of the following questions:

1. Will I follow a path of potential accelerated aging (defined by not engaging in a brain-healthy behavior)?

2. Will I follow a path of potential normal aging (defined by low to medium engagement in a brain-healthy behavior)?

3. Will I follow the High-Octane Brain path (defined by high engagement in brain-healthy behaviors)?

THREE-PATH CHOICE REGARDING YOUR FUTURE BRAIN HEALTH

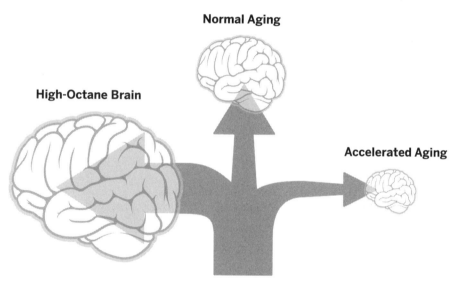

Normal Aging

High-Octane Brain

Accelerated Aging

Figure 2: In any situation, you are presented with a Three-Path Choice regarding your future brain health trajectory.

Occasional or one-time choices are not likely to be consequential for your future brain health. However, your pattern of choices over time significantly influences your brain health trajectory. The more you use the EXCELS Method, the more likely you are to follow a High-Octane Brain trajectory over time and experience the wide range of positive benefits it provides.

Most people already follow the steps in the EXCELS Method to varying degrees. For example, you may reliably engage in optimal amounts of exercise but only inconsistently eat healthy foods. It is not necessary or practical to be perfect across all five of the EXCELS Steps. Rather, the goal is to use the EXCELS Method to help you choose the High-Octane Brain path a little more frequently than you do now and gradually increase the amount of time you spend on that path. Because the High-Octane Brain path creates a positive feedback loop of well-being, you'll be more likely to follow it over time.

MEREDITH AND LOU: GETTING STARTED

Meredith and Lou met a few days before our meeting. They told me they enjoyed their discussion. Meredith looked excited as she described her vision of her Ideal Future Self, which involved a visualization of herself working happily in her garden, having accomplished her two *Whys* for better brain health: "lowering the risk of Alzheimer's" and "staying sharp" for her clients. Lou's vision of his Ideal Future Self was of himself working on his car again. Although he had some difficulty deciding on his two *Whys*, he said his meeting with Meredith helped him zero in on them: maintaining his independence so that he wasn't a "burden" to his son, Al, and being more involved with Al and Al's new fiancée. "They're all I have," he said, looking sad.

We discussed the importance of their repeating the Ideal Future Self vision when brushing their teeth. Doing that even for only a few seconds can help create new neuronal pathways in the brain that bring the vision to mind more frequently. Some people also notice that the Ideal Future Self vision starts to appear when they have to make a choice related to brain health, for example, when they are choosing what to eat or what activity to do.

Finally, we reviewed the Three-Path Choice and the idea that every decision we make involves one of three paths, or choices, regarding our brain health. Imagine that before you make a choice, you visualize the three paths. We'll learn more about what choices to make with each of the five steps, but for now you can imagine that the accelerated aging path would be choosing *not* do something healthy, the normal aging path would be choosing to do a low to medium amount of a brain-healthy habit, and the High-Octane Brain path would be choosing to do a higher amount of a healthy behavior.

In the Three-Path drawing (see figure 2 on page 51), the larger brain on the High-Octane Brain path has two meanings. First, it's a visual metaphor for the improved brain health that people experience on the High-Octane Brain path (i.e., the optimal aging trajectory; see figure 1 on page 10) compared with the path of normal aging and accelerated aging. Second, because all brains shrink as we age, especially in older adulthood, we want to minimize the amount of shrinkage. That is what the habits in the High-Octane Brain have been shown to do—not to mention that people with brain-healthy habits also report higher levels of general health, happiness, and well-being. That's why the High-Octane Brain is the more robust path overall. The acronym EXCELS is a quick way to remember the five steps, or lifestyle habits, that keep us on that path.

The daily choices we make are important, but it's the way they add up over time that puts us more on one trajectory than another. On some days our choices may be much more in line with the High-Octane Brain path and on some days they may not, but on most days we tend to make a combination of healthy and unhealthy choices. One thing you might be surprised to see is that you may already be on the High-Octane Brain path for some of the core habits.

What we're aiming to do is increase our brain-healthy habits even by just a little in each of the five areas. An unexpected bonus is that as we move through the steps, the healthy behaviors often start to propel one another. Some people say that they feel like they are "getting into a rhythm" and that it actually feels easier to integrate more steps. That's why we keep moving forward on the steps even when the results are not perfect.

There's one other important difference between the paths: the High-Octane Brain path is the *only* one that leads to the vision of your Ideal Future Self. Even more inspiring is that when you are following the High-Octane Brain plan, your Ideal Future Self actually evolves, often into an even better version than the one you first imagine.

The Ideal Future Self is meant to be a powerful visual reminder of why we want better brain health and also how we imagine we'll feel when we experience it. By pursuing this vision, we not only make it more likely to occur, we experience other things along the way that we can't even imagine now. Those things are likely to make that vision and the reality of what we experience even richer. That's the case because the path itself promotes health. The whole of you becomes greater than the sum of your individual habits.

HIGH-OCTANE BRAIN ACTION PLAN: THE THREE-PATH CHOICE

Revisit Your Ideal Future Self

Just as Meredith and Lou did, close your eyes and reimagine your Ideal Future Self. Try to make the image even more compelling and joyful.

Reflect: Imagine the Three-Path Choice

Imagine the accelerated aging path on your right, the normal aging path straight in front of you, and the High-Octane Brain path to your left.

Now imagine a common situation that impacts your brain health. This might involve what you will eat, how long you will sleep, or what activity you will do, among other possibilities. On your High-Octane Action Plan, in the section titled the "Three-Path Choice" under the "Chapter 3" heading (page 216), write down the situation you imagined.

Next, imagine that before you make the choice you envisioned, you look down all three paths to get a sense of your options. As you envision the paths, remember that the main High-Octane Brain path is the one that leads to your Ideal Future Self and incorporates your Whys for better brain health.

 Reflect: Strengthening Your Awareness

Every time you brush your teeth, continue to reenvision the High-Octane Brain path leading to your Ideal Future Self. This will help you keep top of mind how your choices in the moment have the power to propel you toward your Ideal Future Self.

TOP TAKEAWAYS

1. Rather than waiting for a catastrophic event to make us improve our brain health or for a future medical cure for Alzheimer's, we can experience a mind-set change right now by realizing that proactive lifestyle interventions provide the greatest protection against Alzheimer's.

2. Research on epigenetics shows that we can affect the expression of our genes—in essence turning them on and off—with our behavior.

3. There are three Navigational Forces that direct our brain health trajectory: (1) foundational factors, (2) health-related factors, and (3) lifestyle factors. Lifestyle factors have the

greatest ability to modify the impact of Navigational Forces 1 and 2 and are the inflection point for enhancing a person's brain health trajectory.

4. The EXCELS Method incorporates the five brain health lifestyle factors with the strongest support for improving our brain health trajectory.

5. Every decision involves a Three-Path Choice: to follow the path of accelerated aging, normal aging, or the High-Octane Brain (optimal aging). The High-Octane Brain path not only reduces the risk of Alzheimer's, sharpens memory, and boosts well-being, it also makes us more likely to experience the vision of our Ideal Future Self as a reality.

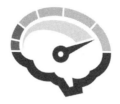

PART II

5 Steps to a High-Octane Brain: The EXCELS Method

"Great things are not done by impulse, but by a series of small things brought together."

—VINCENT VAN GOGH

CHAPTER 4

Step 1: *EX*ercise Is the X-Factor

"Movement [is] a medicine for creating change in a
person's physical, emotional, and mental state."

—Carol Welch

What can a group of bicycling women reveal about the relationship between midlife fitness and the likelihood of later developing dementia in later life? A 44-year-long experiment in midlife cardiovascular fitness was begun in 1968 to find out. One hundred ninety-one Swedish women between the ages of 38 and 60 were classified into three groups based on their peak level of cardiovascular capacity while cycling: a low-fitness group (59 women), a medium-fitness group (92 women), and a high-fitness group (40 women). Among the 44 women who developed dementia, only *2* were in the high-fitness group. *Furthermore, women in the high-fitness group were 88 percent less likely to develop dementia than were women in the medium-fitness group.*

There was also a powerful dose-dependent relationship between fitness level and later dementia such that higher levels (doses) of fitness were related to lower levels of dementia.[80] For example, whereas only 5 percent of the women developed dementia in the high-fitness group, 25 percent of the women in the medium-fitness group developed dementia, as did 32 percent in the low-fitness group. In keeping with this trend, the highest rate of dementia (45 percent) was found in women who could not complete the fitness test because of low cardiovascular capacity. Further, the two women in the high-fitness group who developed dementia were diagnosed on average *11 years later* (at age 90) than were the women in the medium-fitness group (at age 79). As we've learned, even in situations in which dementia may not be entirely preventable, its initial symptoms may be delayed—sometimes significantly—in the presence of healthy lifestyle factors.

The strong relationship between midlife physical fitness level and later dementia was all the more compelling because researchers determined that the results were not related to multiple other factors that have been shown to influence the risk of dementia, such as smoking, drinking alcohol, high blood pressure, and high cholesterol. Although we can't interpret these findings as proof that dementia is caused by differences in fitness level (there are also differences in genetics, diet, or unknown factors to consider), the results are similar to those of other longitudinal studies that have found a dose-dependent relationship between fitness level and dementia.[81] Other studies have similarly shown that the relationship between the two persists even after factoring out the impact of factors that are known to increase the risk of dementia, such as previous strokes and cerebrovascular disease.[82]

Another compelling study showed a 32 percent reduced risk of dementia in adults age 65 and over who exercised three times a week compared with those who exercised fewer than three times per week.[83] A study that pooled the results from 17 other studies showed that the people in the highest-level exercise group had a 38 percent reduced risk of dementia compared with those in the lowest-level exercise group.[84] Also, men age 71 to 93 who walked more than two miles a day had an incredible 77 percent lower risk of Alzheimer's than did those who walked less than a quarter mile a day.[85]

 Hundreds of studies show that physical exercise is related to a reduced risk of dementia and increased volume in brain regions related to memory, attention, and mental flexibility 3.[86]

The positive link between exercise and increased brain volume and cognitive functioning can be seen quite quickly. For example, older adults showed improved memory, mental flexibility (fluidity of thought), and executive functioning and more efficient use of brain networks after just 12 weeks of exercise.[87] Those who engaged in aerobic exercise (in which breathing and heart rate are increased) for just six months showed increased brain volume in several regions of the frontal lobes and in white matter tracts compared with those who did nonaerobic exercise.[88]

"PHYSICAL FITNESS IS NOT ONLY ONE OF THE MOST IMPORTANT KEYS TO A HEALTHY BODY, IT IS THE BASIS OF DYNAMIC AND CREATIVE INTELLECTUAL ACTIVITY."

—JOHN F. KENNEDY

Some studies show that exercise is so effective that it is linked to healthy brain changes many years later. Adults age 65 years and older who walked six to nine hours a week had larger brain volumes nine years later and a reduced risk of developing mild cognitive impairment and dementia.[89] In another study, higher levels of physical activity were associated with reduced levels of beta-amyloid (the protein involved in Alzheimer's) 13 years later and those lower beta-amyloid levels were related to lower rates of cognitive impairment.[90]

How exactly does exercise contribute to protective brain health benefits? Although several mechanisms are involved, one of the most amazing discoveries is that exercise is a core driver of *neuroplasticity*, a process that enhances the physical structure and function of the brain, primarily through a growth hormone called brain-derived neurotrophic factor (BDNF). You'll learn more about BDNF in the interview with Dr. Kirk Erickson, an expert on exercise, brain health, and Alzheimer's (see pages 64–70).

THE MARVEL OF BRAIN PLASTICITY

In 1839, Theodor Schwann proposed that all body tissue is composed of cells, the smallest structural and functional units of an organism. But it wasn't until 1891—when technological developments allowed for greater microscopic visualization—that it was discovered that the brain has its own discrete cells, or neurons. It was presumed that people and animals were born with all the neurons they would ever have and that neurons gradually died over time. This theory changed abruptly in 1962 when, to the shock of the scientific community, it was discovered that animals can grow new neurons. A year later, in 1963, neurogenesis was shown for the first time in human adults. However, as with many revelations that counter established science, it would take another 35 years or so—until the late 1990s—for neurogenesis to be widely accepted in scientific circles.

In business, a 10× change is a point in time when the magnitude of change increases abruptly and profoundly, at approximately 10 times the previous rate, spurring rapid progress and discovery. The late 1990s began a period of 10× change in neuroscience that was galvanized by the growing acceptance of neurogenesis and brain plasticity. Since that time, thousands of research studies have examined neurogenesis in the adult brain.

One of the most critical ingredients for creating new neurons is BDNF, a growth hormone that enhances the physical structure and function of the brain. It functions like a master planner, creating new neurons and rewiring pathways, particularly in the hippocampus.

A 2011 study by Dr. Kirk Erickson and his colleagues is one of the most frequently referenced studies in the field of exercise and brain health and was one of the first to provide support for the powerful relationship between cardiovascular exercise, BDNF, increased hippocampal size, and enhanced memory. Dr. Erickson concluded that loss of hippocampal volume in late adulthood could be reversed with moderate-intensity exercise even if it was started later in life. In the study—a randomized controlled trial of 120 older adults[91]—those who engaged in moderate-intensity aerobic exercise three days a week for one year were able to grow their hippocampus by 2 percent, effectively adding one to two years of volume back to it (the hippocampus shrinks 1 to 2 percent annually in older adults). In addition, those with greater hippocampal growth showed improved performance on a task of visual memory and higher levels of BDNF in blood serum. In contrast, hippocampal volume declined by 1.4 percent in the group that did not exercise.

Although Erickson's study did not prove that BDNF causes increased hippocampal growth, it highlighted that BDNF is a core component of the growth process. It was also notable that those with higher levels of previous exercise showed less hippocampal decline, suggesting that a person's previous fitness level protected against volume loss.

As shown in figure 3 on the opposite page, the increased density of brain tissue in the hippocampi (both the left and the right hippocampus) was not observed in other areas of the brain such as the caudate nucleus (which is related to motor movement) or the thalamus (which is related to sensory processing). This suggests that the benefits of exercise were targeted to the hippocampi, and not randomly occurring in other brain regions. Similar positive changes in hippocampal density after exercise were noted in younger adults ages 20 to 67.[92]

HIPPOCAMPAL GROWTH AFTER CARDIOVASCULAR EXERCISE

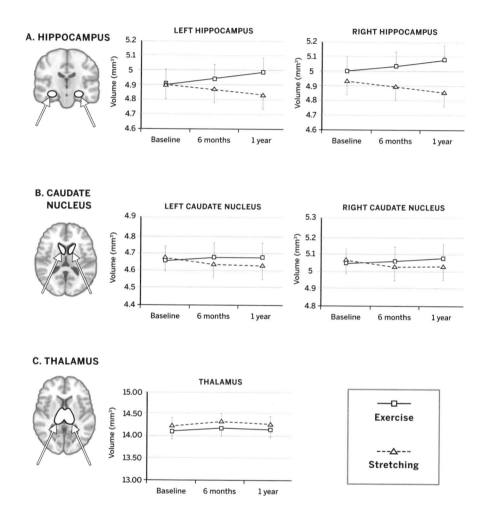

Figure 3: As shown in the top graphs, both the left and right hippocampus showed increased growth 6 months and 1 year after engaging in moderate aerobic exercise three times per week. Hippocampal growth was not shown for the group that did stretching exercises. Cellular growth was specific to the hippocampus, and did not occur in the caudate nucleus or thalamus. Reprinted with permission of the Proceedings of the National Academy of Sciences of the United States of America (PNAS).

Dr. Kirk Erickson on Exercise, Cognitive Function, and Brain Health

Dr. Erickson is a professor in the Department of Psychology at the University of Pittsburgh's Center for the Neural Basis of Cognition. He has received funding from the National Institutes of Health (NIH) for several years and has authored and coauthored approximately 175 medical and scientific articles and 14 book chapters on exercise and cognition.

What is the current state of the science with regard to exercise and brain health?

"If we look closely at randomized clinical trials, we can be confident that engaging in physical activity has a significant impact on a number of different brain health outcomes. One is the effects of exercise on improving some aspects of cognitive function . . . exercise is also a great way of reducing depressive symptoms and anxiety. We are also very confident about the effects of exercise on sleep and sleep behavior. To the extent that all of these things can be put into a bubble that we call 'brain health,' we can be pretty confident that exercise is a very effective way of improving these types of outcomes."

How would you recommend people begin the habit of exercise?

"There are several recommendations I like to give people. One is to think about going slowly, especially in starting up a physical activity regimen. If you want to be physically active, don't try to jump in saying 'I'm going to start running an hour a day' if you're not a runner and if you haven't been running. Work your way up to that hour. Think about it as a long-term goal. You can start by saying, 'I'm going to go for a really good brisk walk for 10 minutes today.' If you're going from not doing anything up to that 10 minutes and do that not just one day but do that for a week or two, then say, 'Okay, I'm going to not do just 10 minutes;

"EXERCISE INFLUENCES EVERY ORGAN SYSTEM IN THE BODY."

I'm going to do 15 minutes.' Each little incremental increase is decreasing the amount of time that you're inactive, and that's really the key. And you're getting yourself in shape, you're not hurting yourself, and you're developing a program, a regimen, that is able to be maintained.

"The other thing that I always tell people is to make sure that you're choosing activities that you enjoy. I can say to myself, 'Oh, I should really start eating more broccoli.' But if I hate broccoli, then it's going to be difficult for me to do that. I might need to find alternative ways of making the broccoli appeal to me more. And it's the same thing with exercise. Here's a personal example: I can say to myself, 'I know that swimming is an excellent activity for me,' but in reality I hate to swim. So by forcing myself to go to the pool, I'm probably not going to be maintaining that type of behavior if I'm not enjoying it."

Is there anything that's been shown to help maintain exercise?
"A buddy system works really well for a lot of people. For example, if you have a plan to meet your friend down in the park to go for a brisk walk or a run, you're not going to leave your friend there by himself or herself. And a lot of people really get benefits from that, and it helps motivate them to continue to exercise.

"On the flip side, there are some different personality types that may be a bit more introverted, that much prefer to exercise by themselves. And this is the time they can actually 'check out' and not have to be engaged in social situations. This is actually my case, for example. For me, exercising is a time when I put my headphones on and I ignore the rest of the world going on around me. Find what works, then fit that into your routine and make sure you stick with that."

Is there an optimal amount of exercise people should do to maximize brain health?
"The physical activity guidelines that were established in 2008—which led the way for the American College of Sports Medicine and the

American Heart Association and all these other guidelines and were also adopted by a lot of other countries around the world—they put the minimum at 150 minutes [per week].

"We went back and reevaluated that for several reasons. One is that there are data, for example, that 75 minutes of activity is sufficient for changing some outcomes in Type II diabetic patients, so you can certainly see benefits at lower doses. The main point is that it's not that you don't see any benefits at less than 150 minutes. It's not like there's a threshold of 150 and then that's when you start to really realize the benefits.

"We also thought about this in terms of the psychology of people who are wanting to get active. What we want to avoid is saying, 'What you should be trying to achieve is 30 minutes per day of activity,' and a person saying, 'Oh, my day is just too busy. I am not going to be able to achieve 30 minutes today, so instead I'm just not going to do anything.' In reality, even if they do 10 minutes, they're getting something from that 10 minutes."

Are you saying there's no "best" way to engage in or maintain exercise?

"That's exactly right. Each person is different, each person likes different things, each person has different barriers they have to overcome. There's the person who says, 'Well, I don't have the time to exercise or go to the gym.' But then you put a treadmill in their house and they still don't exercise. That barrier is not just the transportation to the facility, because they're still not using the treadmill at home. That's clearly not the barrier, so [the solution] is identifying what the barriers are and being true to yourself, being honest with yourself and saying, 'What is it that is not working here? And what's a good way of trying to resolve that?'

"And I think a lot of our technology has been very useful that way. For example, I have a treadmill at home. And in general, I hate running on the treadmill unless I have something to do or something that I can engage myself with. So I have an iPad, I have a Netflix account, and I can watch a fun show, and one hour goes by really quickly on the treadmill then. So it's finding what works and what helps to engage the behavior."

What if someone is already a regular exerciser and wants to use exercise to take their brain health to the next level?

"Unfortunately, we don't have a very good answer at this point. We know that the effects cannot be truly linear. You can't just keep getting smarter and smarter the more you exercise, right? There's got to be a point where there's a plateau. And a lot of it might be dependent on where you're starting out. For an example, let's say somebody's already exercising 200 minutes a week and says, 'What will I gain by going up to 230 minutes a week, 250 minutes a week, or even doubling it? Let's say I'm going to do 400 minutes this week.' If the person's already getting that amount of activity, the improvement or the increase of going up to 250 or 300 or 400 minutes per week might be very, very small, might be absolutely negligible, might not be anything at all. And then also, there might be a point at which you're starting to hurt yourself. You're not just not seeing the benefits, you're doing yourself harm. We certainly have data from other areas in which too much exercise could be potentially dangerous."

You've studied the effect of brain performance related to acute bouts of exercise. What did you learn?

"We can really enhance the way we think; we can really enhance the way that we are learning material, focusing on the material, remembering the material down the road. We get less distracted after we've exercised. So I think an acute bout of exercise can really go a long way. If you avoid physical activity [before an important event], that could also impair your performance. So taking time out instead of thinking of these things as taking up time [is important]."

What about people who begin exercising much later in life?

"I think it's very important for somebody who hasn't exercised in their life to understand that it's not futile for them to start to exercise. They can still, even in older adulthood, achieve benefits. They can still show changes in cognition even if they've been inactive or not exercising for most of their life.

"However, we do really think that the benefits of exercise require maintenance over a long period of time. The earlier you start in life, the better the outcomes are going to be. . . . People who tend to be active earlier in life are also the people that tend to maintain that and be active later in life. It's kind of like developing that habit. And in this case, it's a good habit instead of a bad habit. I really think that trying to engender these types of behaviors in younger populations and earlier in the life span is really important not just for brain health as an outcome but also for just maintaining that behavior."

Is there anything you have seen people become excited about regarding exercise, whether it's a new way to exercise or thinking about exercise in a new way?

"Yes, there's a growing focus on more alternative forms of activity—generally referred to as 'alternative'—like yoga and tai chi . . . a lot of people really enjoy them. And it also adds some mindfulness and relaxation components to it.

"I also think that 'exergaming' has become more and more of a focus of interest for a lot of people—games that try to get people more active. . . . There's somewhat mixed evidence for them being really effective, but I think that part of the reason is that they don't maintain activity for a long period of time. So if you play a game for 30 minutes, you're not active for the full 30 minutes. And then also, most of the interventions have been relatively short in duration. And so I think there are some potential reasons why there's some muddiness right now in that literature, but I think it is a way of getting people active in their living rooms that can be entertaining and kind of fun to engage in."

Do you think some of the less-studied areas such as resistance training and yoga have good support from a brain health perspective?

"Yes, most of the literature right now is on aerobic activities. There's less on some of these other areas. When I reviewed the yoga literature, there are some benefits. And actually, interestingly, some of the effect sizes are about the same as that found from aerobic activities. That being said, the field is just not as mature. There's a mixture of some really poorly designed and conducted studies and some others that are done really quite well. So I think that adds to the instability or the lack of an actual consensus about the effects of yoga or tai chi. There's enough studies out there that I'd say there's certainly something going on, but we just need more work to really be a bit more conclusive about it.

"Resistance training is a really newer area. The field just isn't as mature. And so I think that there's a lot of work that needs to be done, but the work that has been done is pretty promising. And some of the animal work with strength training also suggests possibly different mechanisms by which resistance training influences the brain, that different brain areas or different areas of cognition might be affected. There's a fair amount of work on resistance training and anxiety symptoms. There are certainly gaps in this literature as well, but I think we can be a bit more conclusive that resistance and strength training does impact mood and depressive symptoms and anxiety."

Is there anything I haven't asked you about that you think would be important for people to know as they strive to enhance brain health?

"Not to end on a negative note, but as I said, it's not necessarily a magic bullet just in the sense that if you exercise all the time, it doesn't mean that you won't die from a heart attack. But will it reduce the risk of some conditions and increase the likelihood that you will be performing better and sleeping better, thinking better? 'Absolutely' I think is the answer.

"The other thing is, as we've been talking about, don't give up. It's easy for people to have ambitious aims. We all have our New Year's resolutions, and then people don't maintain them. And there's a reason why people don't maintain them. They think that after starting an exercise regimen, two months from now I'm going to be fitting in these jeans that I can't fit in anymore. So the answer is having goals but being realistic about what those goals are and where you're going to be in a few months' time. These things don't happen overnight, and it takes time and dedication and identifying the barriers. Try to keep going, find things that you enjoy. Those are the real key components, I think, here, to maintaining the behavior."

 The powerful, wide-ranging positive benefits of exercise for the brain and body and the rapid measurable impact of exercise on brain structure and function are why I refer to exercise as an X-factor and recommend that it be the foundation of your High-Octane Brain plan.

HIGH-OCTANE BRAIN ACTION PLAN: EXERCISE

 ### Reflect: Identify Bonus Benefits to Physical Activity

What else do you hope to gain from becoming or staying active besides stronger brain health and a reduced risk of Alzheimer's? Do you want to be slimmer, be stronger, feel more confident, have better balance, maintain your independence, and feel and look healthier overall? Keep in mind what you spontaneously identified and then take a look at the "Bonus Benefits to Physical Activity" table, opposite, for a snapshot of research-supported benefits associated with physical activity. You may be surprised at the myriad ways in which physical activity enhances health, mood, and functioning. Circle all the benefits you want to achieve.

Bonus Benefits to Physical Activity

BRAIN STRUCTURE	Enlarged hippocampus, white matter tracts (facilitating attention and processing speed[93]), overall brain volume[94] Angiogenesis (new blood vessel formation), improved small vein integrity,[95] increased synaptic plasticity/connections between neurons[96]
BRAIN FUNCTION	Stronger memory, learning, attention, processing speed, cognitive flexibility,[97] working memory,[98] perceptual and motor skills
CELLULAR AND METABOLIC CHANGES	New neuronal growth,[99] improved immune functioning,[100] circulation,[101] insulin signaling Decreased inflammation and cellular aging throughout the body,[102] decreased beta-amyloid-related cellular changes[103]
OTHER CHANGES	Improved sleep, mood, mobility, independent functioning, quality of life, metabolism, skeletal function and bone health; weight loss Decreased risk of Alzheimer's, cardiovascular disease (stroke and heart disease), high blood pressure, diabetes, high cholesterol, obesity, all-cause mortality, cancer (bladder, breast, colon, endometrium, esophagus, kidney, lung, and stomach), musculoskeletal pain, risk of falls and fractures, depression, anxiety, and disability

Now pick the top three benefits you circled and write them on your High-Octane Action Plan on the bottom of page 216. It may not be easy to select only three (especially if you circled the whole table, as I did), but picking three helps you bring them to mind more easily, particularly when motivation wanes.

Reflect: Choose Activities That Bring You Joy

Which physical activities bring you the greatest joy? Circle them on the Movement Matrix chart below (or add them if they are not listed). The left column of the matrix includes low-impact activities that can be done with gentle movements to minimize joint pain and chronic pain. Those activities also don't require high levels of cardiovascular endurance. The right column includes activities that can be performed at various impact levels (low to high), depending on your preference. Each of the activities is followed by letters that represent characteristics on which the activity is explicitly focused (defined by the key at the bottom). For example, though all physical activities involve balance, only those which explicitly aim to strengthen balance are labeled as such. By choosing activities that bring you joy and are a fit for you, you are more likely to continue doing them and thus reap the benefits of better brain health.

MOVEMENT MATRIX

LOW IMPACT		VARIOUS IMPACT LEVELS	
Gentle walking	A, N, P, S	Walking	A, N, P, S
Water walking	A	Running	A, N, P, S
Water aerobics	A, R, S	Hiking	A, B, N, P, S
Swimming	A, N	Swimming	A, N
Gardening and yardwork	A, N	Biking	A, N
Yoga	B, F, M, N	Dance	A, B, F, M, S
Tai chi	B, F, M, N	Tennis	A, C, M, N, S
Pilates	B, F, R	Racquetball	A, C, M, S
Bowling	A, C, M, S	Basketball	A, C, M, N, S
Golf	C, M, N, S	Football	A, C, M, N, S
Weight lifting	R	Interval training	A, R
Cross-country skiing	A, B, N, S	Weight lifting	R
Biking	A, N, S	Martial arts	A, B, C, F, M
		Skiing	A, B, N

A = aerobic, B = balance, C = competitive, F = flexibility, M = mental/cognitive activity incorporated explicitly into movement, N = nature, P = pets may easily be involved, R = resistance/strength training, S = social

Under the "Chapter 4" section of your High-Octane Brain Action Plan on top of page 217 write down the top three activities that bring you joy. See if referring to the name of the activity itself (e.g., dance, swimming) makes you more likely to do it than referring to it as "Exercise."

Any Intensity of Physical Activity Is Beneficial

Even though there are consensus guidelines to improve brain health with moderate to vigorous activity, most adults don't exercise nearly enough.[104] Therefore, it's important to note that light-intensity physical activity such as gentle walking is also associated with significant brain benefits.[105] Compared with people who averaged less than 5,000 steps a day, those who walked 10,000 steps a day or more had approximately 1.75 years less brain aging as measured by higher brain volumes. Beyond that amount, each additional hour of light-intensity physical activity a week was linked to higher total brain volumes equal to 1.1 years of decreased brain aging.[106] These findings dovetail with other studies showing that a physically active lifestyle involving tasks such as gardening, housework, and other activities involving bodily movement can also be beneficial to brain health and decrease the risk of dementia.[107]

Immediate Exercise Boosts Are Win-Win

Although there is a positive dose response to brain health with increasing amounts of physical activity,[108] multiple benefits have been noted after just 10 minutes of exercise. In fact, 10 to 15 minutes of moderate-intensity physical activity is linked with short-term benefits in cognitive performance and functional brain changes.[109] Even less than 10 minutes can be beneficial. For example, the 2018 Physical Activity Guidelines for Americans noted that "there is no threshold that must be exceeded before benefits begin to accrue."[110] The guidelines also noted, "A single episode of moderate-to-vigorous physical activity can improve sleep, reduce anxiety symptoms, improve cognition, reduce blood pressure, and improve insulin sensitivity on the day the activity is performed."[111] Some studies have even shown that memory can be enhanced when information is studied either directly before or directly after exercise.[112]

 A 10- to 15-minute Immediate Exercise Boost is a great option if you are pressed for time, are just beginning to exercise, or want to strategically sharpen your memory and attention before special events, meetings, or other functions.

HIGH-OCTANE TRACKER STEP 1: <u>EX</u>ERCISE

 ## Tracking Phase 1

Estimate how many minutes you will engage in physical activity over the next week and jot that down in the "Weekly Exercise Goal" section at the bottom of the High-Octane Tracker (this is just an estimate and may change during the week). Here are a few guidelines to follow:

A. For adults of all ages, strive for *22 minutes a day* (or 150 minutes a week) of moderate-intensity aerobic exercise (or just *11 minutes a day* or 75 minutes a week of vigorous intensity exercise).[113] This level of exercise is associated with a strongly reduced risk of Alzheimer's and a decreased rate of cognitive decline.

B. Start at your current activity and intensity level and build from there only as recommended by your medical provider. Light physical activity (walking) and engagement in active tasks (gardening, household projects, etc.) also count toward your activity minutes. *Any activity is better than no activity*, and even a few minutes of activity can be beneficial to brain health.

C. Additionally, do muscle strengthening/resistance training activities two days a week[114] and balance training for adults over age 65.[115] More health benefits are noted for adults who engage in 300 minutes of moderate-intensity aerobic exercise a week or 150 minutes of vigorous-intensity physical activity (though that level is optional).

 Tracking Phase 2

Record your daily activity minutes on the High–Octane Tracker as follows:

1. In the grid on the bottom left of the High-Octane Tracker, fill in the number of minutes you participated in the activity, followed by the letter L, M, or V to signify the intensity level of the activity as defined below:[116]

   Light intensity (L) = able to sing during an activity
   Moderate intensity (M) = able to talk but not sing during an activity
   Vigorous intensity (V) = cannot say more than a few words without pausing for a breath during an activity

2. Shade in your activity minutes on the High-Octane Brain Diagram (see example on page 78) on a daily basis (and see your "octane level" rise throughout the week, which means you're getting more brain-boosting benefits). The diagram is split into 10-minute increments that total 150 minutes. For light and moderate activities, shade in the same number of minutes you recorded in the grid on the bottom left. For vigorous activities, shade in double the minutes you recorded (e.g., 20 minutes of running = 40 minutes shaded in).

MEREDITH AND LOU: EXERCISE TRACKING

"I have to tell you I was very surprised that exercise is linked to a bigger hippocampus and a bigger brain. I totally need that," Meredith said. "I had no idea!"

"Can't we just take a pill for that?" Lou said, laughing. "I'm just wondering how I'm going to make it all work. I can't move around like I used to . . . probably because I need to lose some weight," he added, patting his stomach.

"Well, maybe that could be one of those Exercise Bonus Benefits that we learned about. You're mainly exercising for better brain health, but maybe you'd also lose some weight? And maybe you'd feel happier?" Meredith asked.

"Maybe. But I can't walk fast, so I don't know how I'm going to exercise for 150 minutes a week," Lou said. "It's not going to happen. I can tell you that right now. The doc said I could follow this program, but I'm not an athlete."

These are the types of concerns that sometimes lead people to stop the process of habit change before they even get started. In fact, the majority of people who exercise, or do "physical activity"—which is a term that can be helpful to use if "exercise" sounds too daunting—are not athletes. Also, most people don't exercise for 150 minutes a week, especially at the beginning. Yes, that is a goal we are aiming for, but it takes time to get there. The beauty of physical activity is that even if you do it for only a few minutes a week, you get brain health benefits. You also can do a variety of physical activities such as working around the house or gardening. With this step and all the other steps, just doing them even a little bit more than you are now equates to progress, especially compared with not engaging in any activity.

Lou agreed to try exercising 10 minutes a day and was surprised that he could start at that level. He said his neighbor was in the hospital and her son had asked if Lou could walk her dog. He seemed excited about it but then questioned how only 10 minutes of exercise a day could make a difference.

It's important to expect that the process of change will be gradual. As long as you are making even one small change, you are moving in the right direction. In fact, the word "OCTANE" is an acronym that reminds us of that. It stands for "**O**ne **C**hange at a **T**ime **A**ccomplished **N**ow equals **E**xcellence." Then you can start stringing together those moments. You don't have to do it perfectly.

Meredith said she'd decided to do the Immediate Exercise Boosts—the 10- to 15-minute bouts of acute exercise—during her lunch hour. She was especially excited that Immediate Exercise Boosts are linked quickly to stronger memory. She hoped that exercising at lunch would help her remember the details of her conversations with clients. She also discussed her excitement about the Bonus Benefits of exercise, noting that she was most interested in slowing her overall aging, improving her immune system, and making her bones healthier. "I had no idea exercise did all that," she said.

We turned our attention to the High-Octane Tracker, since this would be the first week in which they would begin to use it. I recommended that they make copies of the Tracker before filling it out for the first time so they could use it repeatedly. We reviewed an example of how the tracking diagram would look if 70 minutes of exercise was completed in one week (see figure 4 on page 78). The date box at the bottom of the sheet shows that 20 minutes was completed on Tuesday at a light level of intensity (abbreviated with an L), 30 minutes on Thursday at a moderate level of intensity (abbreviated with an M), and 20 minutes on Friday, also at a light level of intensity. Each day, the same number of minutes is shaded in on the brain diagram, which is a visual metaphor for the octane level, or the amount of benefit, that exercise provided to the brain.

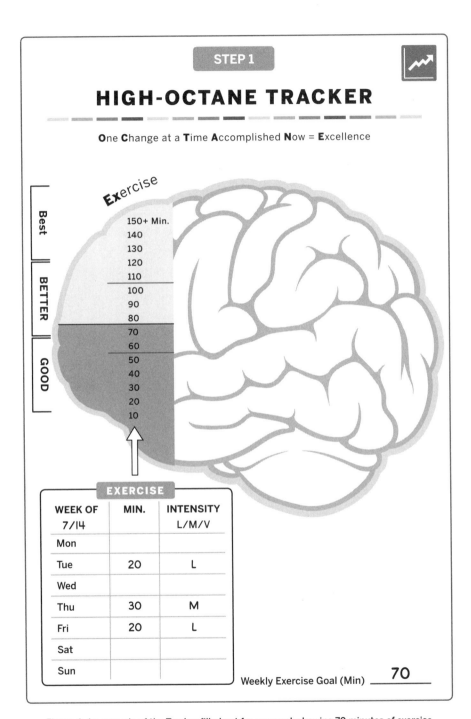

Figure 4: An example of the Tracker filled out for one week showing 70 minutes of exercise completed, and at what intensity.

TOP TAKEAWAYS

1. Exercise is linked not only to a decreased risk of Alzheimer's and decreased age-related shrinkage of brain tissue but also to improved memory, attention, mood, and sleep, among many other benefits. A growth hormone in the brain, BDNF (brain-derived neurotrophic factor), plays a key role in the brain-related benefits of exercise.

2. Although 150 minutes of moderate-intensity exercise a week is recommended (just 22 minutes per day), *any* amount of exercise is beneficial to brain health. In fact, Immediate Exercise Boosts (10- to 15-minute bouts of exercise) have been shown to improve memory immediately and are a great choice to boost cognitive performance before important events.

3. To make exercise a lasting habit, start slowly and build up your routine over time. Consider exercising with a friend or in a class if social support is a motivator for you. Also remember to choose activities that bring you joy (see page 72) so that you are more likely to continue doing them.

4. The Bonus Benefits of exercise are the plethora of positive changes that result from exercise beyond enhanced brain health and a reduced risk of Alzheimer's. Many people find that identifying Bonus Benefits such as weight loss, decreased overall aging, enhanced immune functioning, and better sleep, among many other factors (see page 71), increases their motivation to exercise.

5. Exercise is the *X-factor*, or foundation, of your High-Octane Brain plan because of the strength of the research and the

consensus recommendations showing its significant link to brain health compared with other lifestyle behaviors.

6. Remember that any positive change, no matter how small, brings you closer to having a High-Octane Brain. The acronym OCTANE (*O*ne *C*hange at a *T*ime *A*ccomplished *N*ow equals *E*xcellence), which is printed on your *High-Octane Tracker*, will remind you of this.

CHAPTER 5

Step 2: Consume Healthy Food

"Our bodies are our gardens, to the which our wills are our gardeners."

—WILLIAM SHAKESPEARE

Food has been used to enhance health for thousands of years. In ancient Greece and Rome, food was used to balance the body, prevent sickness, and improve mood. Today, food is often used to promote heart health, treat diabetes, reduce inflammation, boost energy, and manage a host of medical conditions. However, finding accurate information about the relationship between food and brain health is surprisingly difficult. An increasing number of "brain health" diets are based on little or no science, and there is often conflicting information about what to eat for better brain health.

Even though only 31 percent of adults follow a diet to enhance brain health, a whopping 91 percent would be encouraged to do so if they knew more about it.[117] Thankfully, decades of research have converged to provide specific guidance about what to eat—and what not to eat—to significantly reduce the rate of Alzheimer's and slow the rate of cognitive aging.

THE MAP STUDY

In 2004, Dr. Martha Clare Morris and her team from the Memory and Aging Project (MAP) at Rush University began a 10-year study of Chicago residents that looked at the relationship between diet, brain health, and Alzheimer's. The results were powerful and provided specific guidance on how to use diet to enhance the trajectory of brain health.

The participants in MAP completed neuropsychological tests that assessed memory, attention, and other cognitive functions over time. To determine which type of diet might be best for brain health, Dr. Morris and her team calculated scores for how closely the participants followed the Mediterranean diet, the DASH diet, or the MIND diet.

- *The Mediterranean diet* involves high consumption of vegetables, fruits, whole grains, olive oil, and legumes; moderate consumption of dairy products, seafood, and alcohol; and low consumption of sweets and red meat. In the 1950s, it was discovered that the Mediterranean diet was associated with enhanced cardiovascular health. Since then, many studies have supported that link, including a randomized controlled trial—PREDIMED (*Prevención con Dieta Mediterránea*)—that showed an impressive 30 percent reduction in cardiovascular disease among older adults at high risk for cardiovascular compromise as a result of a history of high blood pressure, high cholesterol, smoking, or obesity or a family history of premature coronary heart disease.[118] In 2004, when MAP began, there was already evidence that heart disease and Alzheimer's have common dietary risk factors.[119] Studies have since shown that the Mediterranean diet is linked not only to improved cognitive functioning[120] but also to a reduced risk of Alzheimer's.[121]

- *The DASH (Dietary Approaches to Stop Hypertension) diet* incorporates high consumption of fruits, vegetables, and low-fat dairy foods; moderate consumption of fish, poultry, whole grains, and nuts; and low consumption of saturated fat, red meat, and sweets. The DASH diet, created in the 1990s, is a powerful tool for reducing high blood pressure. It is also associated with a reduced risk of Alzheimer's.[122] Several studies of both the Mediterranean diet and DASH diet support the increasing realization that what is good for the heart is good for the brain.

The main differences between the two diets is that the Mediterranean diet emphasizes high consumption of healthy fats (olive oil), includes wine, allows fewer servings of sweets, does not include a daily recommendation for dairy foods, does not emphasize reduced sodium intake, and is lower in red meat consumption than the DASH diet.

- *The MIND (Mediterranean-DASH Intervention for Neurodegenerative Delay) diet,* developed in 2015 by Dr. Morris and her team,[123] was based on their research from the Chicago Health and Aging Project (which analyzed dietary patterns and cognitive functioning in over 10,000 residents age 65 and over) and the MAP study. Although the Mediterranean and DASH diets weren't specifically created to enhance brain health, the MIND diet was designed expressly for that purpose. The MIND diet includes modified elements of the Mediterranean and DASH diets in addition to foods that have been shown to be neuroprotective in several research studies. Although the Mediterranean, DASH, and MIND diets are all plant-based and low in saturated fats, red meat, and sweets, the MIND diet includes a few notable differences:

- The MIND diet recommends two or more servings of vegetables a day, including one green leafy vegetable (compared with four or more servings of vegetables per day in the Mediterranean and DASH diets, with no specification of type).

- Specification of berries as the recommended fruit two or more times a week (compared with three daily servings of fruit in the Mediterranean and DASH diets, with no specification of type).

- Seafood at least once a week (compared with six or more servings a week in the Mediterranean diet).

- No recommendation for adding dairy foods (which are emphasized in the DASH diet).

- The MIND diet also uniquely recommends limited consumption of five foods—red meat, butter, cheese, fast and fried food, and pastries and sweets—that are associated with accelerated brain aging and a higher risk of Alzheimer's.

The results of the MAP study showed a powerful link between the MIND diet, brain health, and Alzheimer's. For example:

- People who followed the MIND diet at the highest levels of adherence over the course of 10 years (obtaining MIND diet scores in the top third of the group) had a *7.5-year slowing of their cognitive aging* compared with people with scores in the lowest third of the group.

- People in the top third of the MIND diet scores over the course of just four years had a *53 percent reduced risk of developing Alzheimer's* (similar to the results for the Mediterranean diet).

- People with scores in the middle third of the MIND diet scale still had a *35 percent reduced risk of developing Alzheimer's,* showing that even partial compliance with the MIND diet was associated with strong benefits. Conversely, there was no reduced risk of Alzheimer's for the Mediterranean and DASH diets in participants with scores below the top third of their respective scales.

- The MIND diet was *nearly twice as strong in protecting against cognitive decline* as the Mediterranean diet or the DASH diet.

- Green leafy vegetables such as spinach, kale, and collard greens were associated with the slowest rates of cognitive decline. People who ate them about once a day (six or more times a week) over the course of 10 years had a rate of cognitive decline equivalent to that of someone 11 years younger.

- Berries were also uniquely powerful. People who ate berries had a rate of cognitive decline equivalent to that of someone two to six years younger. Furthermore, people who ate two or more servings of berries a week were *52 percent less likely to develop Alzheimer's over five years during the study.*

- Other studies have found that higher adherence to the Mediterranean, DASH, and MIND diets is associated with less cognitive decline and a lower risk of Alzheimer's; the strongest associations have been found for the MIND diet.[124]

What made the results of the MAP study so compelling was that the reduced risk of Alzheimer's was not related to several other factors, including age, sex, obesity, physical activity, education, or history of stroke, diabetes, or high blood pressure. In other words, the level of adherence to the MIND diet in and of itself was a powerful predictor of whether an individual would develop Alzheimer's. Both the Mediterranean and DASH diets have been shown to enhance cognitive functioning in randomized controlled trials, which allows us to say confidently that diet was a causal factor in improved cognitive functioning.[125] The MIND diet is being evaluated in a randomized controlled trial that will run until 2021, at which time we will know much more about the direct cause-and-effect impact of the MIND diet on cognitive functioning.

Available research on the MIND diet has been so compelling that the Alzheimer's Association has chosen to use the MIND diet in the national U.S. POINTER clinical trial, which, like the FINGER study, will test whether multicomponent lifestyle interventions reduce the risk of dementia, but this time in the United States. U.S. POINTER (the U.S. Study to Protect Brain Health through Lifestyle Intervention to Reduce Risk) is also part of a global consortium—called World Wide FINGERS—of similar studies in Singapore, Australia, Sweden, Finland, France, Germany, China, and the Basque region. Importantly, the diet and exercise recommendations may be different for each country (culturally specific), with the goal of providing region-specific brain health strategies. Investigating culturally specific diets is a relatively new line of inquiry in the area of brain health, and World Wide FINGERS is on the cutting edge of this movement.

 A brain-healthy diet slows the rate of cognitive aging and significantly reduces the risk of developing Alzheimer's.

MIND Diet Components

The MIND diet was developed in 2015 and is linked to a significantly reduced risk of Alzheimer's and a decreased rate of cognitive aging. It includes 10 brain-healthy foods and limited consumption of five "brain-deflating" foods.[126]

Daily

- *Six or more servings of green leafy vegetables per week* (the darker the leaves are, the more brain-healthy nutrients they contain).

- *One or more servings per day of other vegetables* (especially cruciferous vegetables such as broccoli, cauliflower, and cabbage, as well as other nutrient-dense options, including carrots, asparagus, celery, onions, mushrooms, zucchini, and sweet peppers).

- *Three servings of whole grains per day* (nutrient-dense whole grains include quinoa, brown and wild rice, oats, cornmeal, popcorn, millet, and farro, among others).

- *One glass of wine per day* (wine type is not specified; research on the cognitive benefits of resveratrol—a compound with antioxidant properties that is present in very small amounts in red wine—has been done primarily in animal studies).

- *Olive oil* is the primary oil.

Weekly

- *Five or more servings of nuts per week* (especially walnuts but also other nutrient-dense nuts such as almonds, cashews, and pecans). If you are allergic to nuts, check with your medical provider about potential substitutes.

- *Four or more servings of beans and legumes per week* (nutrient-dense legumes, including black beans, chickpeas, edamame, lentils, tofu, and lima beans).

- *Two or more servings of berries per week* (nutrient-dense options, including blueberries, blackberries, acai berries, raspberries, and strawberries; fresh berries provide greater amounts of nutrients such as flavonoids than frozen berries; berries are the only fruit recommended in the diet).

- *Two or more servings of poultry per week* (including chicken and turkey, preferably without the skin and not fried to reduce saturated fat).

- *One or more servings of seafood per week* (nutrient-dense options such as salmon, shrimp, sardines, scallops, herring, lake trout, and squid).

NOTE FOR VEGETARIAN DIETS: A combination of grains, vegetables, and legumes produces the "high biological value proteins" that are found in animal foods.[127]

Foods to Limit

The MIND diet also recommends minimizing the consumption of five food groups associated with an increased risk of cardiovascular disease, diabetes, and dementia:

- *Red meats* (aim for no more than three 3 to 5 ounce [85 to 140 g] servings per week; limit saturated fat content as much as possible).

- *Butter and stick margarine* (contain saturated and trans fats; try to consume less than one pat [1.5 teaspoons] per day).

- *Cheese* (a primary source of saturated fat; try to consume no more than 1 or 2 ounces of whole-fat cheese per week;

consider replacing whole-fat cheeses with low-fat cheeses such as part-skim cheeses and cottage cheese).

NOTE: Although there is no consistent evidence on the role of dairy products in dementia risk, low-fat milk and yogurt are recommended to reduce saturated fat intake.

- *Pastries and sweets* (fewer than five servings per week recommended).

- *Fried or fast food* (less than one serving per week recommended to reduce saturated and trans fats).

Beware of Saturated and Trans Fats

Several foods recommended for minimal consumption have high levels of saturated and trans fats. These fats are strongly related to an increased risk of dementia. For example, in the Chicago Health and Aging Project, people who ate more than 25 grams of saturated fat per day had two to three times the risk of developing Alzheimer's over a four-year period.[128]

Saturated fats also are linked to increased levels of *free radicals* (unstable molecules of oxygen that become more chemically stable by binding to other molecules, including brain tissue). Damage from free radicals—oxidation—is a major source of brain aging. We can minimize damage from free radicals by consuming foods that have fewer free radicals (i.e., fewer saturated fats) and more antioxidants. In a sense, antioxidants serve as a decoy for free radicals by binding to them instead of allowing the free radicals to bind to your precious brain tissue.

Dr. Martha Clare Morris on the MIND Diet

Dr. Martha Clare Morris is professor of epidemiology, the director of the Rush Institute for Healthy Aging, and assistant provost of community research at Rush University Medical Center in Chicago. She has more than 20 years of experience studying the relationship between nutrition and the development of Alzheimer's disease and is the lead creator of the MIND diet for healthy brain aging.

Why do you think the MIND diet is associated with a lower rate of Alzheimer's than either of its core components, the Mediterranean diet and the DASH diet?

"The Mediterranean diet is a cultural diet, and the DASH diet was developed for hypertension. The MIND diet was developed to target foods that are related to the brain, so I think it's a more efficient diet that targets the brain."

The top third of people who best adhered to the MIND diet over four years had a 53 percent reduced risk for Alzheimer's. How did that outcome compare with the Mediterranean and DASH diets?

"Those individuals in the top third of scores (the highest level of diet adherence) for both the Mediterranean and MIND diets had similar reductions in the risk of developing Alzheimer's. But the middle category of scores—which was so interesting—was still associated with a 35 percent reduction in risk for the MIND diet only."

What are some of biggest misconceptions about diet and brain health?

"There's this idea that a nutrient you intake from food is the same as taking it from a vitamin supplement, but it's not. There are so many differences. There's also a very common idea that because we've had a series of randomized trials showing that individual vitamin supplements don't prevent dementia, that means nutrition doesn't have anything to do with brain health. But none of the randomized trials done in the United States targeted people who had low or marginal status [levels] of the nutrient. Many of them don't even assess participants' nutrient status at the beginning of the study. If you do a clinical trial and you take everybody who's optimally nutrient-sufficient and supplement them further, you're not going to see an association."

Are there components of the MIND diet that are more challenging than others for some people to integrate?

Dr. Morris indicated that decreasing consumption of pastries is often difficult and that she often tells people: "We're not asking you to give up pastries, but let's see if instead of one serving every day you can cut out sweets on just two days this week."

We also discussed that some people find it difficult to reduce cheese consumption. Dr. Morris recommended reconceptualizing cheese as an accent to a dish rather than eating it in larger quantities. She also noted that leafy greens are sometimes challenging to incorporate "because we're requesting a leafy green serving almost every single day."

What is the impact of tea, coffee, and alcohol on cognitive functioning?

"Tea and coffee... it's just all over the place, with no consistency in the findings.

"Abstainers [from alcohol] have a slightly increased risk of dementia. Those with the lowest risk of dementia have very minimal alcohol intake... seven or fewer drinks per week for a woman [with a comparable intake for men defined as one to two drinks per day]. And with older people, I think it would be closer consumption to that of a woman, because differences in body size and metabolism of foods and alcohol are more similar between older men and older women. And then with each level above very low consumption, you have increased risk."

Research on the Japanese, Nordic, and Argentinian diets shows that some culturally specific foods are associated with brain health. How can we incorporate cultural variables into a brain-healthy diet?

"I have always been concerned that the Mediterranean diet got so much press and attention for prevention of dementia because it's environmentally impractical to be shipping olive oil from Spain or shipping berries to regions of the world that don't have berries. I hope that we can get to a place where we do research in different cultures to find what composition of food and food items is culturally acceptable and environmentally practical to protect brain health."

Could you share how you've integrated the MIND diet into your own life?

"I was on a kick for several years where one of my favorite breakfasts was I would sauté spinach in olive oil and with some mushrooms or onions or red peppers, and then I would have a whole wheat piece of toast, and I would have an over easy egg, and then I would layer it with my leafy greens and squeeze some lemon juice on top of that. So I would have two vegetable servings, one of which was my leafy green serving, right there in my breakfast. And sometimes I would sprinkle some feta cheese in there just for the tang of the cheese." She continued: "This year I was trying to have a leafy green salad for lunch every day. That's a tougher one just because of my schedule and running to meetings two or three times a week."

"I love berries, so that's never been an issue. I have always consumed berries almost every day. I'll have peanut butter toast and I'll smother the top with berries: strawberries or raspberries or blueberries. I also use them as toppings in yogurt, on cereal, and in salads.

"I'm not one of these people who do the same thing every day. I don't do that exercise-wise, I don't do that diet-wise. And so I may have a period of time where I have a habit and then it goes away."

How can people most successfully change their diet?

"Baby steps comes to mind. Manage the goals . . . that's the primary method that our intervention team has used in our clinical trials, a basic behavior modification approach where people identify their goals and what they think they can change in the next week. In the MIND trial, case managers check in with research participants on their goal setting, and ask, 'How'd you do on your goal? What happened when you didn't meet the goal?' And just building on small successes and building the confidence and belief that they can really change."

BRAIN HEALTH SUPPLEMENTS

As Dr. Morris noted in the prior interview, there is no evidence that dietary supplements are beneficial to brain health unless an individual is deficient in a specific nutrient related to brain health. Brain-healthy nutrients should be obtained through a brain-healthy diet rather than through supplements. Similarly, as Dr. Sabbagh noted in his interview (see pages 42–44), the World Health Organization and the National Academy of Sciences have determined that there is insufficient data to support the recommendation of supplements for brain health. Also, a May 2019 survey by the AARP-founded Global Council on Brain Health found "insufficient evidence to recommend any type of supplement for brain health for most adults."[129]

Despite these science-backed recommendations, the use of brain health supplements, particularly among adults over age 50, is on the rise. In 2016, brain health supplements represented a $3 billion global market, and sales are expected to reach $5.8 billion by 2023. The Brain Health and Dietary Supplement survey released by the AARP in June 2019 provided the following insights[130]:

- The most popular brain health supplements include fish oil, omega-3, turmeric/curcumin, and green tea.

- Thirty-six percent of adults over 74 and 25 percent of adults 55 to 73 take a supplement to maintain or improve brain health or to delay or reverse dementia, compared with 23 percent of members of Generation X (ages 39 to 54) and 20 percent of Generation Z and Millennials (ages 18 to 38).

- Seventy-three percent of adults felt supplements could improve brain health, 61 percent believed supplements could delay dementia, and 48 percent believed supplements could reverse dementia.

- Self-reported brain health was no different for those who take or have taken supplements versus those who do not. Healthy eating appeared to be the main factor in higher levels of self-reported brain health.

- Seventy-four percent of the respondents were extremely or somewhat concerned about the effectiveness of the ingredients in supplements, 75 percent were concerned about the purity of the ingredients, and 71 percent were concerned about supplement safety. Forty-nine percent erroneously believed that the supplement industry is regulated by the government through the Food and Drug Administration.

The popularity of supplements is a significant cause for concern. The widespread belief in the effectiveness of brain health supplements provides a false sense of security that frequently costs people precious time and money they might have devoted to strategies to truly enhance brain health and minimize the risk of Alzheimer's. In fact, AARP's Global Council on Brain Health (GCBH) concluded[131]:

Despite claims to the contrary, brain health supplements have not been established to maintain thinking skills or improve brain function. However, there are many other lifestyle habits such as getting enough sleep, exercising regularly, eating a healthy diet, staying mentally active and being socially engaged that are recommended by the council.

The GCBH report[132] also provided important guidance to consumers who might be considering a brain health supplement:

- There is insufficient evidence that multivitamins improve brain health.

- Fatty fish and other seafood may benefit cognitive function, but there is not enough evidence to recommend a fish-oil-derived omega supplement for brain health.

- A deficiency in vitamin B12 or folate (vitamin B9) can negatively impact brain health, and supplementation may be beneficial for people with lower-than-recommended levels. There is insufficient evidence that any other supplements benefit brain health.

- Consumers should be skeptical about brain health supplements because manufacturers often "make vague or exaggerated claims about brain health." In addition, supplements are marketed without governmental review and may contain harmful ingredients.

ALCOHOL AND BRAIN HEALTH

People who drink minimal levels of alcohol on a daily basis (one serving per day for women and one to two servings for men) have slightly lower rates of dementia than do those who abstain from alcohol. This finding has been consistent across multiple studies and is somewhat surprising to many people. One serving of alcohol is equivalent to 5 ounces of wine, 12 ounces of beer (with 5 percent alcohol), or 1.5 ounces of liquor. The protective effect of minimal alcohol use on brain functioning may relate to the connection between heart and brain health, since minimal alcohol use also is associated with the lowest rates of heart disease. However, it is important to note that any amount above that minimal level is increasingly toxic to the brain and is associated with accelerated brain aging. It's important to check with your healthcare provider for personalized recommendations regarding alcohol consumption, especially if alcohol use should be minimized for other reasons and/or there is a history of problems with alcohol.

BRAIN HEALTH DIETS:
ONE SIZE DOES NOT FIT ALL

There is a growing realization that brain health diets differ depending on the foods grown and produced in different geographical locations, in keeping with the dietary practices historically popular with different cultures around the world. Even within the same geographical location, different populations of individuals may have different outcomes from the same diet, suggesting the importance of personalization. For example, both African Americans and white Americans with a parental history of Alzheimer's who followed the "prudent" diet (which emphasizes fruit, vegetables, legumes, fish, and olive oil) had higher cognitive functioning. However, African Americans who followed a "Southern" diet (characterized by fried foods, fats, eggs, organ and processed meats, and sugar-sweetened beverages) had lower cognitive functioning than white Americans who followed the same diet.[133] This is an especially important finding because, as previously noted, African Americans have twice the risk of Alzheimer's as white Americans.

It's also notable that the FINGER trial utilized the Nordic diet, which includes locally sourced foods from Norway, Finland, Denmark, Sweden, and Iceland and emphasizes high consumption of fruits, vegetables, seafood, and low-fat dairy; moderate consumption of game meats and cheese; rare consumption of red meats; and elimination of sugar-sweetened beverages, processed meats, and fast food.

Brain health benefits also have been noted in the Japanese and Argentinian diets,[134] especially in foods containing polyunsaturated fatty acids and antioxidants compared with foods with saturated fats and trans-fatty acids. In light of the ongoing studies associated with World Wide FINGERS, we will soon have much more information about the best culturally specific brain health diets in Singapore, Australia, Sweden, Finland, France, Germany, China, and the Basque region.

NUTRIENTS IN ACTION: THE FUEL-FUNCTION CONNECTION

Understanding how the food and drink we ingest lead to a cascade of specific immediate cellular reactions can help us be smarter about what we're eating. Sometimes the fuel-function connection is more top of mind when we choose gas for our car or food for our children or a pet than for ourselves and own brains.

Most of us have experienced firsthand how quickly substances such as alcohol and caffeine can affect cognitive and motor function. But how does what we ingest impact our cognitive functioning and the physical structure of the brain?

Stage 1

The substances we ingest are broken down by stomach acid and absorbed into the walls of the blood vessels that line the small intestine (some substances, such as alcohol, may be partially absorbed directly into the bloodstream through the stomach; this is why they can affect cognitive functioning so quickly).

Stage 2

These substances are then transported through the bloodstream, filtered by the liver, and transported throughout the body, including to the brain. The brain is a hungry organ; in spite of its relatively small size, it takes in about 20 percent of the nutrients we consume. Neurons absorb some of the substances through a complex filtering process in the capillaries called the blood-brain barrier. That barrier acts as a fortress and is formed by tightly packed cells within capillaries that let only specific substances in, thus protecting brain tissue from infections and toxins.

Stage 3

Neurons use the substances we ingest to perform a variety of tasks, including the following:

A. *Producing neurotransmitters.* Neurotransmitters are the chemical substances the brain uses for different functions, such as movement and memory. For example, choline—which is found in eggs and soybeans—is a building block for the neurotransmitter acetylcholine, which is involved in memory and is the main "fuel" in the hippocampus.

B. *Creating new fats and proteins* from the portions of fats and proteins we ingest. These new fats and proteins are used to make myelin (a fatty substance that acts as a coating to protect neurons) and to grow new connections between neurons, among other functions.

C. *Helping chemical reactions occur.* Vitamins are central to the process of helping enzymes (catalysts for chemical reactions) do their job.

Certain nutrients in food also carry out specific brain functions. Some of these fuel-function connections are depicted in the chart below.

NUTRIENTS AND PHYSIOLOGY

NUTRIENT (FROM FOOD)	PHYSIOLOGICAL FUNCTION IT IMPACTS
Omega-3 fatty acids	Strengthens cell membranes, blood-brain barrier, and neuronal transmission; decreases inflammation
Anthocyanin (an antioxidant)	Strengthens hippocampus and memory (in animal models); found in berries and other fruits
Vitamin E	Potent antioxidant in cell membrane; protects against oxidative injury by binding with free radicals; decreases beta-amyloid deposition, DNA damage, and neuronal loss
Vitamin C	Antioxidant in blood plasma; restores vitamin E
Folate	Builds new DNA and cells

In addition to its direct effects on the brain, nutrition affects brain functioning by altering cardiovascular functioning (healthier diets minimize plaque formation in blood vessels and promote better circulation) and inflammation levels. Inflammation is typically a helpful immune process that is triggered by the body after an injury, but it can become chronic in the presence of high blood sugar, high low-density-lipoprotein blood cholesterol, obesity, and abdominal fat. In addition, the gut microbiome—a bidirectional system between the gut and the brain that is influenced by lifestyle factors—is an emerging area of research connected to Alzheimer's in relation to possible future therapies.[135]

 A healthy diet enhances brain structure and function, improves cardiovascular functioning, and decreases inflammation.

CONNECTING DIET AND CELLULAR ABNORMALITIES IN ALZHEIMER'S DISEASE

A healthy diet has not only been shown to decrease the risk of developing the memory problems associated with Alzheimer's[136] but also the *cellular abnormalities* (tau and beta-amyloid) associated with that disease. For example, multiple studies have shown that high blood sugar levels are related to increased Alzheimer's cellular abnormalities, whereas an "Alzheimer's-protective" dietary pattern (such as the Mediterranean diet) was associated with reduced cellular abnormalities.[137] Further, a recent review of 26 studies showed that adherence to a brain-healthy diet is linked to decreased oxidative stress, inflammation, and accumulation of beta-amyloid and a decreased risk of Alzheimer's.[138] The link between diet and Alzheimer's is so compelling

> "LET FOOD BE THY MEDICINE, AND MEDICINE BE THY FOOD."
>
> —HIPPOCRATES

that the National Institute on Aging–Alzheimer's Association guidelines highlight the direct relationship between diet and changes in brain structure and activity.[139] The guidelines also note an interactive effect among brain-healthy foods, meaning that combinations of brain-healthy foods such those in the Mediterranean, DASH, and MIND diets had stronger health benefits than do nutrients in individual foods.[140]

Reflect: Benefits of the MIND Diet

Review the benefits experienced by people with scores in the top third of the MIND diet scale (on page 84). Then turn to the "Your Desired Benefit from the MIND Diet" section under "Chapter 5" in your High-Octane Action Plan (page 217) and write down your desired benefit(s) from the MIND diet. (For example, some people are more motivated by the idea of slowing their rate of cognitive aging than by reducing the risk of Alzheimer's.)

HIGH-OCTANE TRACKER STEP 2: CONSUME HEALTHY FOOD

Optimizing your MIND diet score is one of the most powerful ways to enhance your brain health trajectory and reduce your risk of Alzheimer's. The steps below are designed to help you do that. Using the MIND diet scoring grid on pages 221, 223, 225, and 228 in your High-Octane Tracker (example shown on page 100), tabulate your score over the next week, based on what you eat. The first 10 rows of the scoring table include healthy foods to incorporate more of, and the last five rows include foods to minimize. Track your food daily by putting a hash mark on the left side of the "Diet Component" column each time you eat a serving of the specified food. Then add up the hash marks in each row at the end of one week, circle your total servings in one of the three columns to the right, and look at the column heading to determine your "weekly points" for that "diet component." (If you eat four servings of green leafy vegetables in one week, your weekly points for that diet component would be 0.5, for example.) At the end of the week, calculate your "Weekly MIND Diet Points" by adding each of the 15 diet component Weekly Points Scores. Your total Weekly MIND diet score will range from 0 to 15. The score during your first week can serve as a baseline score for comparison as you improve your adherence to the diet over time.

MIND DIET COMPONENT SERVINGS AND SCORING

DIET COMPONENT	0 MIND POINTS	0.5 MIND POINTS	1 MIND POINT	WEEKLY POINTS
GREEN LEAFY VEGETABLES	<2 servings/wk	>2 to <6 svgs./wk	>6 svgs./wk	
OTHER VEGETABLES	<5 servings/wk	5 to <7 svgs./wk	>1 svg./day	
BERRIES	<1 serving/wk	1 svg./wk	>2 svgs./wk	
NUTS	<1 serving/mo	1 svg./mo to <5 svg./wk	>5 svgs./wk	
OLIVE OIL	Not primary oil		Primary oil used	
WHOLE GRAINS	<1 serving/day	1–2 svgs./day	>3 svgs./day	
FISH (NOT FRIED)	Rarely	1–3 svgs./mo	>1 meal/wk	
BEANS	<1 meal/wk	1–3 meals/wk	>3 meals/wk	
POULTRY (NOT FRIED)	<1 meal/wk	1 meal/wk	>2 meals/wk	
WINE	>1 glass/day or never	1 glass/mo–6 glasses/wk	1 glass/day	
BUTTER, MARGARINE*	>2 T/day	1–2 T/day	<1 T/day	
CHEESE*	7 + servings/wk	1–6 svgs./wk	<1 svg./wk	
RED MEAT AND MEAT PRODUCTS*	7 + meals/wk	4–6 meals/wk	<4 meals/wk	
FRIED FAST FOODS*	4 + times/wk	1–3 times/wk	<1 time/wk	
PASTRIES AND SWEETS*	7 + servings/wk	5–6 svgs./wk	<5 svgs./wk	

* = Foods to minimize   Weekly **MIND** Diet Points ⇨

Reproduced with permission from Dr. Martha Clare Morris

MIND Diet Component Servings and Scoring

1. After you compute your Weekly MIND diet score, shade in the corresponding "octane" level on the High-Octane Tracker. You'll notice there are now two columns on the tracking system—one for "*Exercise*" (which you continue to fill in as you exercise through the week) and one for "*Consume*" (Healthy Food), where you will shade in your Weekly MIND diet score. These columns allow you to track the first two steps in the five-step EXCELS Method. The "good, better, best" labels outside the brain diagram roughly coincide with the following score groups:

A. Top third MIND diet scores = 8.5 to 12.5 (any score above 8.5 is in the top range; note that the top score of 12.5 represents the highest score that was achieved by participants in the MAP study).

B. Middle third MIND diet scores = 7 to 8.

C. Bottom third MIND diet scores = 2.5 to 6.5.

Tips for Success

1. *Substitute brain-healthy foods into your favorite recipes.* One of the fastest ways to integrate brain-healthy foods into one's diet is to experiment with different ways to prepare the dishes you already enjoy. For example, if you like to make pasta with meatballs, you might experiment with using a pasta made from whole grains, quinoa, or beans and make the meatballs with turkey or tofu rather than beef (add a side spinach salad and you've got your serving of green leafy vegetables for the day). Many cookbooks provide suggestions for making tasty, healthy alternatives to favorite recipes.

2. *Make meal preparation fun.* Because you're more likely to eat unhealthy foods when you are stressed or running late, preparing meals ahead of time can promote healthy eating regardless of the situation that arises. Cooking a few times a week or freezing

seasonal foods is a time-efficient way to integrate brain-healthy foods into your daily routine. Make food preparation fun by playing music, spending time with loved ones while cooking, and cooking at a time when you have few other demands. Pay attention to how you feel when you eat food you've prepared in advance (often there's a positive feeling that creates momentum to do it again).

3. *Cultivate small shifts.* It is natural that the transition to a brain-healthy diet (or any diet) will occur in fits and starts and that on some days it will be much easier to eat healthy than it is on others. Similar to fitness, long-term progress often depends on maintaining small changes over time rather than making large changes that are less likely to be maintained. Build on your successes. For example, you might choose one healthy food you'd like to incorporate more of and aim to increase it by one or two servings in the next week (thankfully, the MIND diet requires fewer servings of many foods than the Mediterranean and DASH diets, so it's easier to meet recommended amounts). Continue to increase your servings by one or two each week only if you were successful in increasing your servings the week before.

   You also might consider choosing one of the five unhealthy foods (see page 100) to decrease and try to decrease your usual number of servings by 25 percent (e.g., if you eat fried food four times a week, try eating it three times a week). If you're up for a major challenge, see if you can stay below the recommended weekly serving listed for at least one of the unhealthy foods. But whatever approach you take, make sure that it grows by small shifts and that you add a new change only after you've consistently incorporated the previous one.

MEREDITH AND LOU:
HABITS ARE HARD TO BREAK

"I couldn't believe it, especially after only 10 minutes of exercise, but it happened again two more times this week!" Meredith exclaimed. She was beaming as she recalled feeling sharper and more productive on each of the three afternoons when she had exercised the week before.

Many people are similarly surprised at the rapid cognitive benefits of 10- to 15-minute Immediate Exercise Boosts and use them strategically to enhance attention and memory before important events. Those sessions also promote better sleep, improve mood, and lower blood pressure.

Meredith often homed in on the immediate benefits of brain-healthy habits. She wanted to see the improvements as soon as possible and knew that doing that would motivate her to make brain health a part of her life. In fact, some people are able to achieve their weekly High-Octane Brain exercise goal simply by doing a daily Immediate Exercise Boost, creating a win-win scenario for short-term and long-term brain health.

Lou already had noticed an improvement in his sleep that resulted from increasing his physical activity. He'd walked his neighbor's dog, Daisy, twice the week before and felt he slept more soundly on those nights. This was especially important to him because he usually didn't feel well rested. However, he also expressed concern when recalling something his wife had mentioned to him a few times: "She said my snoring got to her. I tried to use different pillows, but it didn't seem to help." We discussed the idea that sometimes the combination of snoring and not feeling well rested could be a signal of a sleep-related problem. Lou agreed to mention it to his doctor.

Lou also showed us his High-Octane Tracker. "I did better than I thought . . . I'm at the 'Good' level," he said, pointing at the Exercise column, which had 43 minutes shaded in. He was surprised that he was able to count walking Daisy as exercise because he had so much fun doing it. I can't stress enough that the more enjoyable a physical activity is, the greater the likelihood is that it will become part of your lifestyle. The good news is that all five EXCELS steps can—and should—be tailored to be enjoyable. The goal for the next week was for Meredith and Lou to maintain the level of exercise they had done the previous week and, if possible, increase it by five minutes.

We also reviewed the highlights of the MIND diet in preparation for the second step of the High-Octane Tracker (**C**onsume Healthy Food), which they would begin that week. The light gray columns on the brain diagram are tracked and scored on the pages that follow the diagram, and the white columns are tracked directly on the diagram itself. For example, "Exercise" is a white column and is tracked directly on the diagram, and "Consume Healthy Food" is a gray column and is tracked on the next page. The scores are added up weekly, and the total score is shaded in as the octane level in that column.

"And then at the end of the week, just make sure all of your octane levels are filled in on the brain diagram," Meredith noted, looking at Lou. "It's like an at-a-glance comparison of which of your habits are stronger than others. Then you can compare your progress week to week by just glancing at the differences."

"But I'm eating the wrong things," Lou said, looking down. "I'm a meat-and-potatoes guy. That's how I was raised. So all this talk about vegetables and stuff . . . I don't even know how to cook." Lou explained that his son Al and Al's fiancée Rachel had been preparing many of his meals since his wife died.

"Maybe you should show Al and Rachel the MIND Scoring System and see if they can start to bring you foods from the MIND diet," Meredith suggested.

We also discussed that prepared foods at grocery stores can be healthy, tasty alternatives for people who don't cook. Green leafy vegetables are especially powerful: six servings per week is linked with an 11-year slowing of cognitive aging over 10 years. (And though 10 years was the length of the study, continued benefits after 10 years seem likely, though this needs to be quantified.)

Meredith said she had started to "hide" vegetables in a variety of foods, including casseroles and smoothies. "My husband says he hates vegetables, but he never even notices them," she said, laughing.

TOP TAKEAWAYS

1. The Mediterranean diet, DASH diet, and MIND diet all promote brain health.

2. Compared with the Mediterranean and DASH diets, the MIND diet is twice as effective at protecting against cognitive decline and reduces the risk of Alzheimer's even with only partial dietary compliance. People who followed the MIND diet at the highest levels for four years had a 53 percent reduced risk of Alzheimer's, and people who followed it at medium levels had a 35 percent reduced risk.

3. Culturally specific diets are being studied and may expand options for brain-healthy foods.

4. Even though brain health supplements are not effective except in cases in which an individual is nutrient-deficient, 73 percent of adults believe that supplements can improve brain health, and the industry for brain health supplements is projected to reach almost $6 billion by 2023.

5. Green leafy vegetables and berries are especially powerful in reducing the rate of cognitive aging.

6. Nutrients reach the brain through the bloodstream and help neurons carry out many important functions.

7. A healthy diet improves brain structure and function, enhances cardiovascular functioning, reduces inflammation, and decreases Alzheimer's-related cellular abnormalities.

8. You can enhance your brain health by identifying which benefits of the MIND diet are most important to you and optimizing your MIND diet score.

CHAPTER 6

Step 3: Engage and Learn

"Learning is a kind of natural food for the mind."

—Cicero

So far we have focused on ways to maximize the trajectory of our brain health with exercise and nutrition. But what about the way we use our brains to engage and learn? Can that optimize our brain health trajectory and reduce our future risk of Alzheimer's? Amazingly—and powerfully—it can.

Remember the SuperAgers, the Fabulous Four, and the individuals from the Rush Memory and Aging Project (MAP) (see pages 81–85) who didn't express the symptoms of Alzheimer's even though they had Alzheimer's-related cellular abnormalities? A common denominator among all those groups was a high level of engagement in activities.

The benefits of engagement have been explored in dozens of studies. One type of engagement with particularly strong support for minimizing the risk of Alzheimer's is cognitive leisure activities. Such activities include reading, playing games, playing a musical instrument, and other activities that people engage in for enjoyment or well-being[141] and that require active information processing. In several studies, higher levels of engagement in cognitive leisure activities was linked to a significantly lower risk of Alzheimer's[142] and—as noted in the MAP study—a reduced likelihood of expressing Alzheimer's symptoms even if related cellular abnormalities were present. Researchers have recommended that memory-preserving activities should begin in middle life and continue through later life.[143]

THE POWER OF COGNITIVE RESERVE

How could involvement in activities enhance future brain functioning? One theory suggests that engagement promotes higher levels of *cognitive reserve* (increased neuronal capacity). Higher neuronal capacity means that the brain communicates in a more efficient, flexible way.[144]

 Cognitive reserve refers to increased neuronal capacity, communication, and efficiency. Higher levels of cognitive reserve are linked to a significantly lower risk of Alzheimer's disease and a delayed expression of Alzheimer's symptoms if related neuronal abnormalities are present.

The power of cognitive reserve has been shown in several studies:

- In the Chicago Health and Aging Project, people who participated in activities such as reading, playing games, listening to the radio, and viewing television only once a year to several times a year were twice as likely to develop Alzheimer's as people who engaged in such activities several times a week.[145] A different study showed a 2.6 higher rate of Alzheimer's in people who were cognitively inactive than in those who were most active.[146]

- In an analysis of over 29,000 people across 22 studies, participation in mentally stimulating leisure activities was associated with a 50 percent reduced risk of developing Alzheimer's.[147]

- Higher cognitive engagement was also associated with a reduced risk of mild cognitive impairment, a potential early form of Alzheimer's.[148]

- An analysis of 19 studies across different cultures found that mentally stimulating leisure activities were associated not only with a reduced rate of cognitive decline but also with better memory, speed of processing, and executive functioning/mental flexibility.[149]

- In a 44-year-long study of over 800 women, those who engaged in more cognitive tasks involving the arts, intellectual information, or religious components had a significantly lower risk of Alzheimer's.[150]

HOW CAN COGNITIVE ENGAGEMENT BE MEASURED?

There is no single best way to measure cognitive engagement, as the scales and methods used vary by research study.[151] Among the available measurements, the Cognitive Activity Scale (CAS) that was used in the Bronx Aging Study[152] provides a weekly measure of cognitive engagement that is most easily applied to the weekly High-Octane Brain tracking format.

In the Bronx Aging Study, 469 participants age 75 and older were followed for up to 21 years with detailed clinical and neuropsychological evaluations that looked at the relationship between cognitive engagement and later dementia. At the beginning of the study, the participants rated their frequency of participation in six activities: reading, writing, crossword puzzles, board or card games, group discussions, and playing a musical instrument. They received one point for each "activity day" they participated in over the course of the week, with a maximum number of seven weekly points for each activity. For example, if a person read on a daily basis, they received seven points. If they also played card games three days that same week, they received three additional points, for a total of 10 activity days that week.

Astoundingly, participants with CAS scores in the highest third of the scale (more than 11 activity days per week) had a 63 percent lower risk of dementia (including Alzheimer's and vascular dementia) than participants with scores in the lowest third of the scale (seven activity days or less per week). Each one-point increase/additional activity day was associated with a 7 percent reduction in the risk of dementia. Importantly, this association remained strong even after the researchers factored out the impacts of age, sex, educational level, the presence or absence of chronic medical illnesses, and initial cognitive ability. A follow-up study further revealed that each additional activity day delayed the onset of accelerated memory decline by 0.18 year.[153]

In the Bronx Aging Study, reading, playing board games, and playing musical instruments were associated with the lowest rates of Alzheimer's. However, it's important to note that across dozens of studies, no one specific cognitive activity has been associated with a lower risk of dementia. In the Bronx Aging Study and most other studies, there was no measurement of the duration of time in which an individual engaged in the activity, though in light of the types of activities assessed, it can be generally assumed that participation lasting at least 15 minutes was necessary to engage in the activity. The Bronx Aging Study and other studies also considered the possibility that the relationship between cognitive activity and dementia was circular, meaning that perhaps people who already had cognitive impairment were simply less engaged in activities. But even after accounting for that possibility, the relationship between cognitive engagement and future cognitive functioning was robust.

Dr. Yaakov Stern on Cognitive Reserve, Aging, and Alzheimer's

Dr. Yaakov Stern is a professor of neuropsychology at the Taub Institute for Research on Alzheimer's Disease and the Aging Brain and chief of the Cognitive Neuroscience Division in the Department of Neurology at Columbia University Medical Center in New York City. He is internationally recognized for his research in cognitive reserve, aging, and Alzheimer's disease and is currently investigating the neural basis of cognitive reserve.

What is cognitive reserve, and why is it so important to brain health?

"There are brain changes that occur with aging or with various conditions like Alzheimer's disease. The idea of cognitive reserve is that given those brain changes, some people will cope with them better than others. There are sets of life experiences that provide people with the ability to do that."

How does the brain function differently for someone with low cognitive reserve versus high cognitive reserve? What's the effect from abnormal cellular changes such as those associated with Alzheimer's disease?

"We've found two things. . . . You can find a 'network,' a set of brain areas that are activated during a task. People with higher and lower reserve might use the same set of brain networks, but those networks might be used more efficiently or with higher capacity in individuals with higher cognitive reserve. Let's say you give people a task that gets harder and harder. What will typically happen is the areas of the brain that are involved in doing that task will increase in activation as the task gets harder. We found, and others have found, that people with higher reserve show less of an increase in the use of those networks, as if those networks are more efficient.

"The example I like to give is, let's say I have to swim and you have a well-trained swimmer from a swim team. If you ask me to swim two laps, I could do it. I'll be huffing and puffing. The well-trained swimmer could do that with ease. That's similar to efficiency.

"When you're studying reserve . . . optimally, what you would want to do is control for the state of the brain. By that I mean that in normal aging without Alzheimer's pathology there are all these things that happen—brain volume shrinks, the white matter might not have the same integrity. So you want to match for all of that because cognitive reserve is not about the brain. It's about the functioning. And then look for differences in activation when doing different tasks as a function of experiences that are associated with cognitive reserve: IQ, education, and occupation."

What is *compensation*? How does it relate to Alzheimer's disease?
"In my definition, *compensation* is when you start to use other sets of brain areas that you don't typically use. You can say, 'Okay, you're compensating for a difficulty, perhaps age-related changes or Alzheimer's-related changes,' so you reach out to some different brain areas. That's compensation, the way a cane is compensatory. What we see very often is that people with higher reserve don't have to reach out to those other areas. Those other areas really are not as good as the primary areas, but if you need to use them, at least you can do the task. Like when you have a cane, you can still walk, but you can't run like you could if you didn't use a cane.

"But a lot of other people, when they think of compensation, they think of it where it allows you to do better. That's possible as well. So perhaps in certain cases you reach out for another way to do it or an extra set of brain areas that allow you to do the task better. There have been people publishing showing that those who compensate in specific tasks actually do better on those tasks.

"We're talking about task-related activation, which is specific to one task or another. Another concept is . . . if you look at early studies of the onset of Alzheimer's disease, many studies have shown that people with higher education are less likely to develop Alzheimer's disease within a period of time. So the people with higher education can stave off the pathology longer. And when they do that, it's not one task that's benefiting. It's everything . . . memory and day-to-day function, etcetera. So perhaps there are aspects of networks in the brain that are not task-specific that allow us to compensate better or that moderate the effects of pathology better."

> "I'M VERY INTERESTED IN INDIVIDUAL DIFFERENCES AND WHY SOME PEOPLE AGE MORE SUCCESSFULLY THAN OTHERS."

What would you recommend to an older adult who wants to increase his or her cognitive reserve beyond the sum total of his or her life experiences?

"The way I think about it is that reserve is not something that's fixed. So the sum total of experiences throughout the lifetime contributes to reserve. Clearly, people are born maybe genetically endowed with the potential for a certain IQ, at least to some degree. That's very much influenced by early education. Those early experiences clearly are important. But then the data show that occupational experiences make a great difference . . . how stimulating your occupation is cognitively or in other ways . . . [for example] physically. Then we've shown that late-life leisure activities are important. Also, social networks. And those are just what people have studied. There are experiences across the life span that contribute to reserve. So there's no reason to think that experiences acquired later in life wouldn't also contribute.

"When people retire, very often they do more poorly. Sometimes when people retire, they just sort of stop. They don't do their job, but they don't do anything else. And that's no good. It's sort of a complex relationship. . . . The other idea is that perhaps people who retire stay more active, they take advantage of retirement to do the activities that they like to do, remain socially active, be engaged. That's very important."

Has your research influenced the way you manage your own brain health?

"Part of it is easy for me. I feel like I'm very much wrapped up in my work. It's intellectually stimulating. I interact with very smart people. So part of it for me is attempting to continue to do that for as long as I can. So I'm 65. When will I retire? I really like what I'm doing. I would continue it as long as I can get the grants. I work at a medical center, so basically in order to continue to do what you do, you have to get the grants. So that part of it is to maintain the intellectual stimulation and collegial stimulation that I get from my workplace. I'm not in a rush to retire. I'm sure we all know people that are active in their eighties and nineties now. It's a different world.

"Another part . . . [is] exercise. I was never an exerciser. I don't think my parents exercised, and I wasn't raised to think that it was so important. So as I understood that exercise is important, I realized that was something I had to incorporate into my lifestyle. But behavior change is very hard. We moved back from the suburbs into New York City, my wife and I, about five or six years ago, so I walk a lot more. At the hospital, my office is on the nineteenth floor, so every day when I go down to get my lunch from the cafeteria, I walk back up to the nineteenth floor. I try to incorporate that walking into my lifestyle. The other thing that I've done is started to take tai chi. Tai chi is sort of interesting because it has this mindfulness component. Also, it's difficult in terms of balance. I can't tell you I'm a tai chi master. Now, should I do more? Probably. According to recommendations, probably I should be hitting the gym, doing some aerobic exercise, some strength training that I'm not doing. I've done that in spurts, to be very honest. But it's hard for me to maintain that."

What questions would you like to research in the future?
"About eight or nine years ago, I started a whole new study looking at cognitive aging in a very intensive way with all kinds of imaging, both structural and functional, just so I could understand that better. Part of the reason is I want to understand cognitive aging better. But part of the reason is that as I understand what underlies the brain changes and the network changes that underlie cognitive aging, maybe I can apply reserve to it more efficiently."

ARTISTIC AND SOCIAL ENGAGEMENT

Other factors that contribute to cognitive reserve include engagement in social, artistic, and craft–related activities. A 2015 Mayo Clinic study of older adults (average age 87) found that the risk of developing memory problems decreased by 73 percent when people were engaged in artistic activities (e.g., drawing, painting, sculpting) in middle and later life. The risk decreased by 55 percent when people socialized in middle and later life, by 53 percent when people used computers in late life, and by 45 percent when people did craft activities (e.g., woodworking, ceramics, sewing) in middle and late life. Several other studies have also shown that social engagement—including social activities, social relationships, and social support—is linked to improved cognitive functioning[154] and happiness.[155]

In spite of the popular focus on crossword puzzles and brain games, no specific task has been consistently linked to stronger cognitive reserve. It is most important to engage in tasks that are personally appealing to you. Various studies have shown that the following activities are linked to stronger cognitive reserve (in no particular order):

- Reading books and newspapers
- Social engagement (spending time with other people)
- Playing games such as cards and checkers
- Doing crosswords, jigsaws, and other puzzles
- Writing
- Listening to the radio
- Watching television (and actively paying attention to the information)
- Doing crafts (woodworking, needlepoint)
- Visiting museums
- Playing a musical instrument
- Engaging in artistic activities (drawing, painting, sculpting)
- Attending religious services
- Belonging to social clubs
- Participating in discussions with others
- Studying and attending classes
- Learning a new language

In spite of the popular focus on crossword puzzles and brain games, there is no specific task that is best at strengthening cognitive reserve.

OTHER STRATEGIES TO ENHANCE COGNITIVE FUNCTIONING

We know that engagement in leisure activities can enhance cognitive functioning and decrease the risk of Alzheimer's, but what about strategies like brain games and memory aids (mnemonic devices)? Should you incorporate those strategies into your High-Octane Brain plan? Let's consider the different goals of commonly used cognitive tools.

Cognitive *Compensation* Tools

These techniques are designed to help you use your existing memory skills more efficiently in a specific situation (such as learning a person's name) but are not primarily aimed at increasing the capacity of your memory in general. The most popular tools involve techniques to process and remember information effectively. These strategies stem from classic experiments investigating how people learn most effectively and include techniques such as repeating, categorizing similar information together ("chunking"), and connecting information to be remembered with information that is already stored in memory ("linking"). Other compensation strategies promote better ability to pay attention (e.g., removing distractions, taking breaks) and cope with word-finding difficulties. Many people are interested in such strategies to cope with common daily memory problems, or brain blips (see pages 120–25).

Cognitive *Enhancement* Tools

Whereas compensation techniques provide strategies to more efficiently process and remember information in a *specific* situation, enhancement techniques are used to improve underlying cognitive skills, such as memory, across a *range* of tasks. This is similar to the way an athlete might exercise a specific muscle in order to improve the ability to use that muscle in a variety of activities.

There are two major types of enhancement techniques:

- *Cognitive stimulation:* Cognitive stimulation refers to "participation in a range of activities aimed at improving cognitive and social functioning."[156] If this sounds familiar, that's because this is the category for cognitive leisure activities. These techniques often enhance a person's underlying cognitive functioning above and beyond the activity in which they engage.

- *Cognitive training and brain games:* Cognitive training refers to "guided practice of specific standardized tasks designed to enhance particular cognitive functions."[157] This increasingly popular category encompasses brain games and other programs (delivered via computer or in person) that are designed to enhance cognitive functioning through a training program.

DO BRAIN GAMES ENHANCE COGNITIVE FUNCTIONING?

There are few topics in the field of brain health more controversial than brain games, or computerized cognitive training (CCT). One of the reasons for the controversy is that different groups of researchers have come to very different conclusions about the effectiveness of CCT. Those opposing conclusions, along with highly publicized lawsuits alleging false advertising against multiple manufacturers of brain games, have led to significant confusion about the ability of CCT to truly enhance cognitive functioning. The controversy reached a high point in 2014 after the Stanford Center on Longevity published an open letter signed by 70 scientists who concluded that brain games do not offer a proven way to reduce or reverse cognitive decline. The scientists further argued that the best evidence suggested that "cognitive health in old age reflects the long-term effects of healthy, engaged lifestyles."[158]

The Stanford letter concluded that the benefits of CCT were "small" and the effects of doing them did not translate to other tasks beyond the games themselves. This lack of transfer of the learned skill to the real world was considered especially concerning because people often do CCT because they believe it will enhance their overall cognitive functioning and daily abilities, not just their performance on the CCT.

A few months after the Stanford letter, 133 scientists and practitioners issued a statement in which they argued that CCT was effective in enhancing various cognitive and everyday activities. A 2016 study sought to examine these competing conclusions by reevaluating the research considered by both groups. That study concluded that there was "extensive evidence that brain-training interventions improve performance on the trained tasks, less evidence that such interventions improve performance on closely related tasks, and little evidence that training enhances performance on distantly related tasks or that training improves everyday cognitive performance."[159]

Several studies in recent years have continued to show no sustained effect or generalized benefit from CCT, whereas fewer have shown a notable benefit. The best-known of the latter is the Advanced Cognitive Training for Independent and Vital Elderly (ACTIVE) study, which is the first large-scale randomized trial to show that CCT improves cognitive function in older adults. In the ACTIVE trial, training occurred for 10 to 14 weeks initially, with booster sessions thereafter. Benefits to daily functioning and memory were noted 5 years after training,[160] and enhanced daily functioning, reasoning, and processing speed were noted 10 years after training.[161] This made ACTIVE the first major study to show long-term benefits to cognitive skills and daily function. ACTIVE participants were 33 percent less likely to develop dementia over 10 years, and those who completed the most processing speed training (11 to 14 sessions) showed a 48 percent reduced risk of dementia compared with older adults who did not do the training.[162] Other studies have also shown that CCT can improve memory in the short term and long term,[163] and still others have shown CCT to be "modestly effective" at improving cognitive performance in healthy older adults (though that efficacy varies across cognitive skills and is largely determined by training type).[164] Specifically, there is some support for Useful Field of View cognitive training (which examines the speed of visual processing, and is linked with driving ability)[165] and programs used in the IMPACT trial (which showed improvements in general memory and attention skills[166]), among others.[167]

The latest science supports the conclusion that although most commercially available CCT interventions have no consistent scientific support and often do not achieve transfer and longevity of the trained skills, a minority of programs have been shown to effectively enhance cognitive skills in the short term and long term and to promote transfer of those skills to daily life. Therefore, if you elect to use a CCT as part of your brain health plan, it's important to ensure that you're selecting the most effective CCT. To help people navigate this growing market, in 2015 the Institute of Medicine released a report on cognitive health and aging with recommendations for consumers to consider when evaluating CCT options.[168] Look for the following issues to be addressed by commercially available CCTs on their websites or in their program materials:[169]

- *Real-world effectiveness:* Has the product demonstrated that it affects performance on real-world tasks of concern (e.g., the ability to manage finances, medications, and other daily tasks)?

- *Research quality:* Has the product been evaluated by comparing an experimental group with a group that did not receive the same CCT intervention (a control group)? Did both groups include individuals with the same expectations of cognitive benefit?

- *Length of effectiveness:* Does the product demonstrate long-term benefits?

- *Other factors that affect the product's effectiveness:* Are there factors (e.g., age, health, motivation, general cognitive ability) that affect the benefit of the product?

- *Independent verification:* Have the benefits of the product been replicated by independent groups that do not benefit in any way (financially or otherwise) from the research findings?

- *Comparative effectiveness:* Have the benefits of the product been compared to the benefits of other products or lifestyle choices,* such as physical activity, intellectual engagement, social interaction, and diet, that may impact affect cognitive health?

  NOTE: This is particularly important to consider in light of the well-established, significant benefits of the other brain health lifestyle interventions addressed in this book. If you decide to use a scientifically supported CCT, consider doing so only as one of several aspects of your brain health plan.

TIPS FOR BRAIN BLIPS

The following is a roundup of cognitive compensation techniques that can help us navigate the brain blips we all experience from time to time. The first three techniques use a three-step "P-L-R" method that also can be applied to other brain blips that require memory:

1. Pause

2. Link

3. Rehearse

Brain Blip 1: Forgetting the Name of Someone You Just Met

It can be embarrassing to forget the name of a person you just met or the name of an acquaintance you haven't seen for a while. This often occurs when we didn't create a strong, memorable link to remember the name when we first learned it. Here are some steps that can help:

Step 1: Pause and pay special attention to the person's name. Then repeat the name out loud after you are introduced ("Nice to meet you, Robin"). By saying the name out loud, you allow the person to correct you if necessary and create an opportunity to rehearse it, which allows you to better remember it.

Step 2: Link the person's name to someone or something you know well. In most situations, you can link the new name to another person you know who has the same name or a famous person with the same name, but in some cases—as depicted in the drawing below—the new name may be the same as or similar to that of a well-known object. If you are linking the new name to the name of someone you already know, adding an image can help. For example, picture the face of your cousin Robin as you look at the Robin you just met.

Step 3. Rehearse the new name and link you created. After meeting Robin, repeat her name to yourself several times while picturing the link you've created.

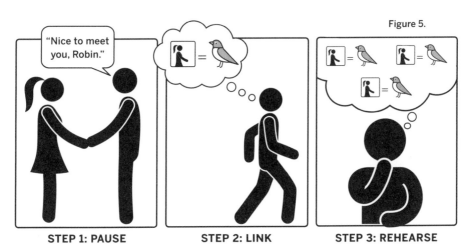

| **STEP 1: PAUSE** | **STEP 2: LINK** | **STEP 3: REHEARSE** |

Brain Blip 2: Misplacing Objects

We are most likely to misplace commonly used objects like keys, glasses, purses, and wallets. This usually happens because we use the objects in multiple settings, often while engaged in other activities that may distract us from remembering where we put them.

Step 1: Pause to place the item in its *home space*—a specific place where you consistently put an object. This includes a hook by the door for keys (as depicted below), a shelf for a purse or wallet, or a dedicated space on a dresser or table for glasses. Make sure your home space is convenient and that nothing else is put in that space so that you're more likely to use it consistently.

Step 2: Link the object to its surrounding area. If you put the object in its home space, this step is generally unnecessary, as you know where it's located. However, in situations where there is no home space or we forget to use a home space, study the visual scene *around* where you placed the object. Notice what room is it in and what surface it's on.

Step 3. Rehearse the location to yourself—while you picture it—at least three times. For example: "My keys are by the back door." Or, if you put your keys in an area that was not a home space, "My keys are on the table in the living room."

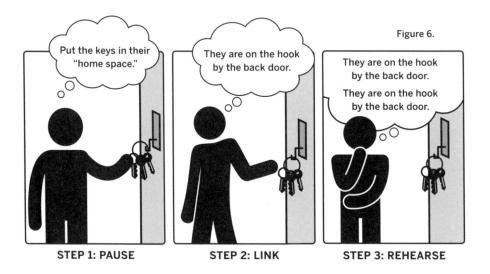

Figure 6.

STEP 1: PAUSE   STEP 2: LINK   STEP 3: REHEARSE

Brain Blip 3: Forgetting New Information

Let's use the following limerick to demonstrate how to use the P-L-R technique when you are trying to learn and remember new information. The same technique can be applied to information you read or hear in conversation.

> *Brain health is the foundation*
> *For all of your creations.*
> *By growing your mind*
> *You will find*
> *Success in your vocation.*

Step 1: Pause and pay close attention to the words as you read them. Reading the words out loud can also be helpful, especially when they have a rhythmic pattern (creating a rhythmic pattern for words that don't inherently have one can also be helpful).

Step 2: Link the words of the poem to mental pictures. For example, you might picture the ground (a "foundation") with the words "Brain Health" written on it to help you remember the line "Brain health is the foundation." Next, you might imagine the word "Create" extending upward from the ground to help you remember the line "For all of your creations." Combining these aspects into a two-part visualization can help you link the first two lines together, particularly if you practice saying the words as you think of the images. To remember the line "By growing your mind," you might imagine that the word "Create" is angled up toward your head, or your "mind," which is linked to "success." Finally, you could picture yourself shaking hands with someone (a symbol for "success in your vocation"). This is just one example of how to use a mnemonic technique. Linking words to pictures is often a very individualized process, so experiment to find whatever helps you remember the limerick most effectively, especially because we will come back to it later.

Step 3. Rehearse the limerick, along with the associated visuals, until you can repeat it three times without error.

Brain Blip 4: Word-Finding Difficulties

Word-finding difficulties occur when we cannot think of the word we want to say. The strategies to manage this tip-of-the-tongue phenomenon are different from the P-L-R technique we just covered.

Figure 7.

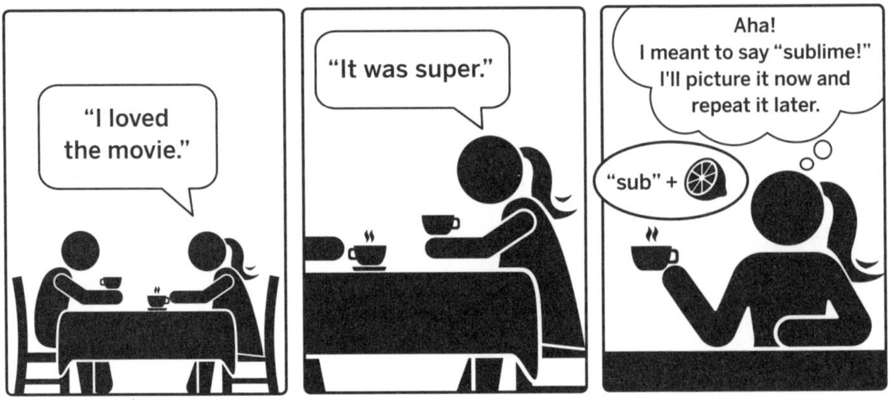

| STEP 1: KEEP TALKING | STEP 2: SUBSTITUTE SYNONYM | STEP 3: REHEARSE |

Step 1: Keep talking. As depicted above, if you stumble upon a word-finding difficulty during conversation, keep talking (rather than pausing to try and think of the word you want to say, which may draw attention to your difficulty and could slow the process of retrieving the word). By continuing to talk, you may activate the neuronal pathways in the same geographic region of your brain where the target word is and retrieve the word more quickly.

Step 2: Substitute a synonym. Let's say you want to say the word "sublime" but cannot think of it in the moment. Try substituting a synonym for "sublime," as depicted above ("super"). If possible, choose a synonym with the same first letter as the target word, because this sometimes helps the target word come to mind more quickly. If you can't think of a synonym with the same first letter, use a generic synonym that begins with any letter (e.g., "terrific" or "great").

Step 3: Rehearse the target word after it comes to mind and pair it with a visual image so that you remember it better (in this case the word "sub" is paired with a picture of a lime to make you remember the word "sublime"). Don't worry if you can't think of the target word for a while. It often comes to mind when you least expect it. But when it does, rehearsing it can bring it to mind more readily the next time you use it. If it doesn't come to mind, you can always describe it to someone else and see if he or she can help you retrieve it. Then rehearse it.

Let's revisit the limerick exercise. Can you recite the limerick without looking back at it? If so, congratulations! If not, repeat the P-L-R technique a few more times and see if that improves your recall.

BRAIN ACTION PLAN: ENGAGE AND LEARN

Congratulations! You've now learned the key ways to optimize brain health by engaging in cognitive activities. We've reached the exciting point of integrating the *E*ngage and Learn step into your High-Octane Action Plan!

Reflect: What Activities Appeal to You?

Write the three cognitive and social engagement activities that appeal most to you in the "Appealing Cognitive Activities" section under the "Chapter 6" heading of your High-Octane Action Plan on page 217. You can identify those activities on your own or by referencing the list on page 115.

Track: Over the next week, make a tally mark in the "Engage" grid at the bottom of the High-Octane Tracker each time you complete a cognitive leisure activity that lasts at least 15 minutes. For example, if you read for 15 minutes on Monday and then did a puzzle for 35 minutes the same day, you would make two tally marks on Monday, signifying that you completed two activities. Then shade in the corresponding octane level for each day and watch the level rise over the week. Because of the way the original research was conducted with the scale on the High-Octane Tracker (and similar scales), additional points are not provided for durations longer than 15 minutes.

Note that you will be tracking the first three steps of the EXCELS Method this week (**EX**ercise, **C**onsume Healthy Foods, and **E**ngage and Learn).

MEREDITH AND LOU: EXPANDING ENGAGEMENT

"He's all I've got, and now I'll barely see him anymore," Lou said softly. "And . . . I shouldn't say this because he's my son . . . but it reminds me of what I don't have." Lou looked as if he'd been crying as he shared the news that Al and Rachel would be moving to California after they got married.

"On top of that," he continued, "my doctor wants me to get tested for sleep apnea. I might as well quit."

We discussed Lou's original motivation for participating in the High-Octane Brain program, how he wanted to be independent as long as possible and continue engaging in his relationship with Al and Rachel at the highest level possible. At moments of difficulty, it can be very helpful to review our *Whys* and our Ideal Future Self vision, which can serve as a touchstone to remind us how to keep our brain health on track.

Lou seemed to be relieved after taking a few minutes to revisit his vision of his Ideal Future Self. He had been working very hard and had to make a lot of progress in a short time, which Meredith reminded him about. She also shared that she'd felt discouraged a few weeks earlier. "What I've learned," she said, "is that even though sometimes we are afraid and sad and lonely, we're here. The only other alternative is not to be here and not to better ourselves in the ways that are most important to us. We are our own best hope for having the future we want."

We later discussed the third step of the High-Octane Brain program: **E**ngage and Learn. Meredith realized that most of her cognitive activity involved her work and seemed excited to add some variety. She spoke of her surprise that artistic activities counted as engagement and explained that she was looking forward to getting reinvolved in painting. She then encouraged Lou to consider spending some time working on his car because that too would count as an engagement activity.

Lou reported that he was having conversations with neighbors when he walked Daisy, something that counted toward his engagement points. Dual activities like this are considered *Multipliers* in the tracking plan and can be counted in multiple categories. (In Lou's case, his walks with Daisy counted as exercise *and* engagement because of his conversations with others while he exercised.)

We finished with a little reminder that engagement activities should be tabulated daily on the grid beneath the brain diagram on the High-Octane Tracker. The corresponding octane level also could be filled in daily (many people find that doing this serves as a visual motivator). Although the top level of engagement activities per week is 11 or more, as with all the other steps, doing any activity is better than doing none. Any time you read, do a puzzle, or have a stimulating conversation—all these things count! You can look back at the list (see page 115) to see the wide range of activities that count. The points add up pretty quickly.

Many people feel that the last three steps—engagement, stress management, and sleep—seem to flow a bit more easily, perhaps because they have more immediate restorative benefits. They also seem to require less effort and planning. Going back to that idea of synergy, the last three steps often bolster progress on the first two steps.

TOP TAKEAWAYS

1. Cognitive reserve (CR) refers to increased neuronal capacity that allows the brain to process information more efficiently. You can increase CR by engaging in cognitive leisure activities, social activities, and arts and crafts. Higher CR is linked to a significantly decreased risk of developing Alzheimer's.

2. Cognitive compensation tools help us use our existing memory more efficiently in specific situations (e.g., remembering a new name), whereas cognitive enhancement tools are used to strengthen underlying memory across a range of situations.

3. Brain blips can be minimized with cognitive compensation techniques such as Pause-Link-Rehearse.

4. Although most online brain games do not show a sustained benefit or generalize to real-world situations, some do. Consumer recommendations are available to help you vet potential options. If you choose to use them, online brain games should be only one component of your brain health plan.

5. In spite of the media focus on crosswords and online brain games, no specific task has been linked to higher levels of CR. Engage in tasks that are personally appealing to you (see page 115 for ideas).

6. People who engaged in 11 or more activities a week as measured by the Cognitive Activity Scale (CAS) had a 63 percent lower rate of Alzheimer's than people who engaged in 7 or fewer activities a week. The numerical targets on the High-Octane Tracker are informed by research on the CAS.

CHAPTER 7

Step 4: *L*ower Stress and Boost Well-Being

"Do not let the fact that things are not made for you, that conditions are not as they should be, stop you. Go on anyway. Everything depends on those who go on anyway."

—ROBERT HENRI

The human body is primed to respond rapidly and effectively to acute (sudden) stressors. Within milliseconds of a potential threat—a loud noise, a child wandering near the street, the unexpected brake lights of the car in front of us—a surge of hormones (cortisol and adrenaline) prepares us to spring into action for safety and survival. However, repeated exposure to stressful situations often wreaks havoc on the body, mood, and brain. Not only does chronic stress increase the risk of cardiovascular conditions such as high blood pressure, heart disease, and diabetes, it is also linked to depression. A growing body of research also shows a strong relationship between chronic stress and Alzheimer's disease.

Consider the following questions about your experiences in the past month:

1. How often have you been upset because of something that happened unexpectedly?

2. How often have you felt that you were unable to control the important things in your life?

3. How often have you felt confident about your ability to handle your personal problems?

4. How often have you felt that things weren't going your way?

5. How often have you felt that you were on top of things?

6. How often have you felt that difficulties were piling up so high that you could not overcome them?

These questions measure your perceived stress level. Stress is our bodily and emotional response to changes and demands and is tightly connected to the way that we interpret situations. Because the answers to these questions have been shown to relate strongly to future cognitive functioning, these items are integrated into your High-Octane Tracker, where you can track—and ideally lower—your scores over time.

The same questions were asked of over 6,000 ethnically and socio-economically diverse people age 65 and older during the Chicago Health and Aging Project. Their answers were compared with their performance on neuropsychological tests over a period of almost seven years. The results showed that individuals with the highest levels of perceived stress had lower cognitive functioning and a significantly faster rate of cognitive decline compared with those with the lowest levels. That connection remained even after the researchers factored out other possible explanations, such as smoking, blood pressure, personality characteristics, and chronic medical conditions.[170] Other studies have shown more rapid rates of cognitive decline among individuals with high lifetime stress levels.[171]

High perceived stress also is linked to lower cognitive performance. For example, in a study of over 1,000 adults age 64 to 100, those with the highest perceived stress had worse performance on several cognitive tasks, including measures of memory, processing speed, verbal production, and attention.[172] Unfortunately, high stress also increases the likelihood of being diagnosed with a cognitive disorder. In over 1,900 adults age 70 and older, those with the highest amount of perceived stress were 30 percent more likely to develop mild cognitive impairment.[173]

One study that included more than 10,000 adults investigated whether midlife stress levels (measured at age 56) were linked with cognitive functioning about 13 years later. The results showed a strong relationship between stress levels and cognitive impairment. Among the more than 1,500 participants who developed dementia, the highest rates were among those who had rated their midlife stress as medium to high many years earlier.[174]

THE LINKS BETWEEN STRESS, DEPRESSION, AND ALZHEIMER'S

Depression can be related to many factors, but chronic stress is a leading cause. Depression is a serious condition that affects more than 300 million people worldwide[175] and is often characterized by feelings of sadness, emptiness, and/or decreased interest in previously enjoyable activities. Depression may also affect a person's thoughts, behavior, bodily functioning, and cognitive functioning. The symptoms may include negative thoughts about and perceptions of the world, including increased pessimism, hopelessness, and worthlessness. Changes in bodily functioning are also common, including increased fatigue, problems with sleep and appetite, and decreased speed of movement and/or speech. Cognitive changes may include decreased concentration, memory, and decision making. Decreased engagement in activities and increased isolation are also common. Clinical depression involves symptoms that last two weeks or longer and so is different from the temporary low mood that many people periodically experience as a result of situational or other stressors. Depression may be chronic, or it may start later in life. In severe cases, it may involve suicidal thoughts.

There is also a powerful, sobering link between depression and Alzheimer's. In an analysis of 23 studies of nearly 50,000 people older than age 50, those who were depressed were 65 percent more likely to develop Alzheimer's.[176] Other studies have shown that people with depression had a 50 percent higher risk of developing Alzheimer's.[177] Unfortunately, it's not clear whether depression causes cognitive impairment or whether cognitive impairment increases the likelihood of depression.[178] Emerging areas of research are examining whether the longevity of depression is a factor in determining the risk of Alzheimer's.[179]

Chronic stress is the most frequently studied cause of depression and is linked to an increased rate of depression and Alzheimer's through factors that are common to both, including the following:

- Altered connections between the body's stress response/ endocrine and nervous systems (via the hypothalamic pituitary axis[180]). For example, high levels of cortisol, a primary stress hormone, are noted in many individuals with Alzheimer's and depression.

- A smaller hippocampus and decreased neuronal growth in the frontal lobe (a region involved in mental flexibility, strategy formation, decision making, and working memory).

- Chronic inflammation, which is linked to reduced repair of neurons and neuronal death.[181]

Studies still need to be conducted to determine whether treatment of chronic stress and depression can minimize the risk of developing Alzheimer's,[182] but there is promising evidence that treatment of depression positively impacts cognitive functioning. First, individuals with mild cognitive impairment with decreased depression had a lower likelihood of developing Alzheimer's than did those whose depression did not improve.[183] In addition, multiple studies have shown that treatment of depression in older adults resulted in improved cognitive function.[184]

Findings like these suggest that treatment of depression can improve cognitive functioning and may help slow cognitive decline after it has developed. Treating depression also offers more immediate benefits to a person's mood and quality of life. Fortunately, there are several methods to treat depression effectively.[185] Most research shows that a combination of antidepressant medication and psychotherapy is more effective than medication alone.[186] Also, reductions in depression of 20 to 25 percent over one to two years are reported after the use of psychological interventions alone.[187]

Treating depression is important beyond its connection to Alzheimer's. Better mood and increased well-being are associated with enhanced cognitive performance.[188] For example, in a study of more than 11,000 adults age 50 and over, those with the highest levels of well-being (characterized by a questionnaire including items such as "I look forward to each day" and "I feel that my life has meaning") had the highest levels of cognitive functioning.[189] However, it's important to remember that the most important (and first) step in treating depression is to discuss it with a medical provider.

AMPLIFIED BENEFITS: PHYSICAL EXERCISE AND MINDFULNESS

Two other interventions also help treat depression but also uniquely amplify the positive benefits of other steps in the EXCELS Method: physical exercise and mindfulness.

Physical exercise and mindfulness boost mood and well-being, minimize depression and stress, improve brain structure, enhance cognitive functioning (sometimes within minutes), and improve sleep (as we'll learn in chapter 8). Another bonus is that they are also associated with decreased cellular aging throughout the body.

1. *Physical exercise:* As we have previously discussed, physical exercise significantly enhances brain structure and function and dramatically reduces the risk of developing Alzheimer's. Exercise also helps decrease the symptoms of depression for many individuals. For example, an analysis of multiple studies that

included over 48,000 people showed that exercise significantly reduced symptoms of depression.[190] Other research shows that the benefits of exercise may be enhanced when it is paired with antidepressant medication.[191]

Happiness is also linked to exercise. A recent review of 23 studies showed that the amount of exercise was a powerful factor: 52 percent of the "very active" group reported feeling happy, compared with 30 percent of the "sufficiently active" group and 20 percent of the "insufficiently active" group.[192] Although the data do not suggest that exercise causes happiness (it's possible that happier people exercise more), knowledge of this connection may provide added incentive to consider exercising, especially if your mood is not optimal. In situations in which motivation is low, it can be helpful to remember that frequently motivation increases *after* we take action.

2. *Mindfulness:* Mindfulness is the practice of paying attention to the present moment in a nonjudgmental fashion. It is associated with a wide range of emotional, cognitive, and physical benefits, including the following:

   A. Decreased worry and improved memory functioning[193]

   B. Decreased depression and anxiety[194]

   C. Decreased cortisol (a stress hormone) in older adults with high baseline cortisol levels[195]

   D. Enhanced hippocampal connections[196] and increased density of brain regions related to memory, emotion regulation, and perspective taking[197]

   E. Enhanced attention, memory, verbal production, and cognitive flexibility[198] as well as decreased age-related cognitive decline[199]

Studies show that meditation (broadly encompassing mindfulness and other practices that involve directed attention and awareness) is linked to improvements in blood levels of beta–amyloid (a biomarker for

Alzheimer's) and improved cognitive function, sleep, mood, and quality of life in adults 50 and older who initially report cognitive decline.[200] Meditation is also linked to reduced cellular aging throughout the body.[201] An innovative study of long-term meditators showed a significantly slower trajectory of cellular aging after age 52. Furthermore, the slowing of cellular aging was directly proportional to the number of years a person meditated,[202] which was theorized to potentially be explained by the positive impact of meditation in reducing chronic stress.

 Physical exercise and mindfulness provide amplified High-Octane Brain benefits. They boost mood and well-being, decrease stress and depression, improve brain structure, enhance cognitive function (sometimes within minutes), and improve sleep. As an added bonus, they decrease cellular aging throughout the body.

Despite the myriad cognitive and structural brain benefits associated with mindfulness, one crucial connection had been missing from recent research until recently. Increased hippocampal growth after mindfulness training, which had been shown in several studies, had never been linked to a change in cognitive functioning.

This changed in 2019 when Dr. Jonathan Greenberg and his colleagues at Harvard Medical School showed that increased hippocampal growth was linked to improvements in working memory (the ability to keep information temporarily in mind while completing a larger goal).[203]

Dr. Jonathan Greenberg on Mindfulness, Brain Health, and Well-Being

Dr. Greenberg is a clinical and research fellow in the Integrated Brain Health Clinical and Research Program of the Department of Psychiatry in Massachusetts General Hospital and Harvard Medical School. He researches the impact of mind-body and mindfulness training on cognitive, emotional, and physical function among individuals with chronic pain, injuries, and depression, among other conditions.

Many people have heard about mindfulness but are not sure exactly what it is. What is mindfulness?

"I typically start by giving the most commonly used definition suggested by Jon Kabat-Zinn: 'Paying attention in a particular way . . . on purpose, in the present moment, and non-judgmentally.' I also find it helpful to convey that you can boil it down to two main components, as proposed by Bishop and colleagues (2004[204]).

"One component is awareness to what's happening now . . . what I'm seeing, what I'm hearing, the sensations of my body. It could be the emotions that I'm feeling now, the thoughts that are running through my head. It could be the words that somebody else is saying to me. It could be the motorcycle that I'm now trying to fix as a mechanic. I could be doing anything as long as I'm paying attention to what's happening now.

"The second component is an orientation of acceptance and non-judgment . . . just allowing it to be as it is. In a nutshell, mindfulness is knowing what's happening now and being open to and non-resistant to it."

How is mindfulness different from meditation or prayer?

"Mindfulness can be a meditation, but it doesn't have to be. You can practice mindfulness by brushing your teeth mindfully, eating mindfully, driving. . . . Some may think that they must sit with their legs crossed and eyes closed and be in this altered state of consciousness in which mindfulness arises. As long as you're in the present moment, rolling with it, trying to allow things to be—you can be mindful by doing anything. Prayer can be a mindful practice, and other types of meditation can involve a mindful component, but mindfulness doesn't have to be a meditation-related practice.

"All of us have mindful moments every single day even though we may not conceptualize them as such—any time we are engaged, interested, curious, and attentive about what's happening now. . . . We've all been mindful. . . . The only difference is the new component of intentionality: 'Let me try to keep my attention on this, and whenever my attention wanders I'll bring it back and I'll try to be kinder to myself. And even if I am tired, even if I am unfocused, I try to be understanding with myself and know that I am trying to cultivate this new intention that my mind may not be used to.'

> "IF YOU'RE WALKING DOWN THE STREET AND THINK, 'THIS SUNSET IS SO BEAUTIFUL,' YOU'RE JUST LOOKING AT IT, YOU ARE WITH IT, YOUR MIND IS WITH IT. THERE'S NO INTERNAL STRUGGLE OR STRIFE, AND YOU'RE JUST ROLLING WITH THE MOMENT."

"For me it's been a profound experience personally to be mindful of not being mindful: 'Oh, I'm totally not focused right now . . . I'm kind of tired. How does that feel? How does my body feel? How does my breath feel? What thoughts arise in my mind when I can't focus and I'm frustrated? Let's try to be curious.' That's the investigative mentality. 'Let's say: Bring it on. Let's have it. That's an interesting experience. How is messiness? What is anger like? Oh, wow, isn't that interesting?'"

Besides the misconception that someone must always feel calm and serene while practicing it, are there other misunderstandings about mindfulness?
"[Mindfulness] still has a connotation of being 'New-Agey,' some would even say 'quack-like.' Over the past few years this stereotype has diminished because there's a lot of evidence and science behind it now. . . . It [mindfulness] doesn't have to include a spirituality component at all . . . it's a practice of attention and awareness and acceptance."

Paying attention in the moment often involves confronting negative thoughts and feelings. How does one stay mindful in the presence of negative thoughts and feelings?

"Some people envision mindfulness as this serene, calm, focused experience. . . . That's one of the primary misconceptions I work with. Mindfulness is the opposite in a way. The ability to be with difficult emotions is a main feature of what mindfulness is. Because our initial tendency—our knee-jerk reaction—is to run away from unpleasantness and get rid of any unpleasant emotion, thought, or sensation. That is how people begin to cultivate avoidance, which is also the hallmark of numerous anxiety-related conditions and is exacerbated by difficulty tolerating discomfort. Mindfulness encourages us to rest and relax into even negative emotions. It can be scary at first because it can be considerably difficult to just be with difficulty.

"Mindfulness may even temporarily increase discomfort in the short term, but with practice, you discover there's a big freedom in being able to be with negative emotions and not have to do anything about it. You don't have to dwell on it. You can realize, 'Yes, it's unpleasant and I'm breathing heavily and I'm sweating and I'm having this thought that is just horrible. But it's okay to feel and think that way. It doesn't mean that anything needs to be done about it. It's a temporary event that arises and passes away. Just like everything else.'"

People often wonder whether negative sensations and thoughts will decrease over time if they allow themselves to experience them. Does that happen?

"It's important to emphasize that the goal is not to reduce negative sensations and thoughts. That is an occasional welcome but transient side effect but not the essence of the practice. Rather, we aim to be with anything that may come our way, be it positive or negative, without having to push it away or cling to it. . . . We cultivate this skill and integrate it into our lives, but there are ups and downs, and no matter how far we think we've come, sometimes we'll spend days ruminating over something entirely silly that happened. And that's expected. It's just the way things go. So if we set expectations for that ahead of time, people won't see it as failure when it does come. And it will come.'"

Sometimes people may not respond to negative experiences in a catastrophic way but may just seem more withdrawn and not as alive. Can mindfulness help increase awareness of joy?
"Certainly. Mindfulness can help us pay attention to, absorb, and be present with positive things as well. This may be particularly helpful for individuals facing mental, emotional, and physical challenges, who tend to be preoccupied with negative experiences. We are hardwired and predisposed to focus on negative events, since they pose a potential threat to our survival. Evolution drives us to preserve our life and pass on our genes and is not as concerned with our emotional well-being and quality of life. But the ability to be aware and accepting of the present moment can also enable us to better recognize and enjoy positive and joyful experiences as well because we're right there with them as they happen and can learn to override the tendency to get back to our pain or negative emotion."

Could you describe how the findings from your 2018 study on working memory inform our understanding of the connection between cognitive functioning and mindfulness?
"Working memory is a cognitive system with limited capacity that is responsible for temporarily holding information. It's actually one of the most crucial determinants of intelligence and higher cognitive functioning because most higher cognitive functions are dependent on working memory. We have to hold the relevant information readily available and utilize it for tasks we need to perform. One of the things I like about that specific study is that there are numerous studies showing that meditation can impact hippocampal function and structure. But what does that mean? How does that relate to people's lives?

"That particular study relates to 'proactive interference,' when old information prevents the learning and remembering of newer information. Where I work, we have to change the passwords for our computers every three months, and everybody keeps entering their old passwords after a recent change. That's one example of proactive interference. The old memory—the old material—interferes with retaining the newer material. And it's crucial that we let go of this older and no longer relevant material in order to be open to what's happening now, open to new material. It is a decoupling of no longer relevant information so we will be open and available to learning something that is happening, something that we may not be used to, but something novel that may be useful for us to carry forward."

Could mindfulness help improve age-related declines in working memory?

"It is possible. In many cases the hippocampus tends to shrink as people get older, and mindfulness may be protective of hippocampal volume. Dr. Sarah Lazar from the Department of Psychiatry at Massachusetts General Hospital is finishing up a big study with older adults, checking whether mindfulness training can stave off cognitive decline and associated functional and structural changes in the brain, and we are anxiously awaiting the upcoming results.

"Some studies [about the impact of mindfulness on cognitive skills] show improvements in attention following mindfulness training, and others show no improvement. Some show improvements in memory, and others do not. But we do know specifically that autobiographical memory can improve, and that's particularly relevant to individuals who are suffering from depression. These individuals sometimes can have difficulty recollecting specific autobiographical memories, and mindfulness can help with that. We do know that it can help with cognitive flexibility. But it's not a blanket overarching way of improving all of your cognitive functioning."

What brain changes have been linked to mindfulness?

"There's not really one singular part of the brain that's the 'mindfulness core.' The amygdala is the part of the brain that has to do with fear processing, anxiety, and threat detection. We know that when people practice mindfulness, once they are confronted with negative stimuli—a negative picture or negative movie clips—their amygdala is less active. Reductions in stress following mindfulness training have also been associated with increases in gray matter density in the amygdala (suggesting possibly more refined emotional regulation). Mindfulness also relates to the hippocampus, which is related to learning and memory. It can counter hippocampal shrinkage, which is common in PTSD [post-traumatic stress disorder] and depression and in people with childhood adversity. Some frontal regions associated with mindfulness have a lot to do with cognitive flexibility, self-control, and higher cognitive function. So there are multiple parts of the brain that mindfulness can target."

What is the best way to learn mindfulness?

"People get involved with mindfulness in different ways. What was helpful for me was to start with a structured course. And that could be Mindfulness-Based Stress Reduction, an eight-week structured group course that's available nationwide, or Mindfulness-Based Cognitive Therapy, a structured program aimed at preventing depression relapse as well as for other conditions. The structure helps with support from the group and from the teacher. You can just Google 'Mindfulness-based stress reduction' and find places near you that offer it.

"There are also intensive meditation retreats—sometimes they're called Vipassana retreats—that could be 7 or 10 days of silence. That's how I started. I found them incredibly beneficial. But not all people can take 10 days out of their lives and families and seclude themselves in this type of training. I would highly recommend it if that's possible. If it's not possible, a mindfulness-based stress reduction course is two hours a week with daily home practice of 40 minutes.

"It can also help to read a book while you do it, such as Jon Kabat-Zinn's *Wherever You Go, There You Are* and *Full Catastrophe Living*. There are also numerous mobile apps that can help with the training, such as Headspace, Calm and Breathe, and others, and they can be useful in making the practice accessible throughout the day. There are also YouTube videos. I would recommend starting with a structured program and a relevant book while sustaining daily practice with the aid of recordings, videos, and apps and independently."

How long do you recommend that people practice mindfulness on a daily basis?

"There's no clear answer. Some studies show that the more you practice mindfulness, the more benefit you get, and others don't show that correlation. It's difficult to say because the people who choose to or are able to practice more may be inherently different from those who do not. They could possibly be more gritty; maybe they have more drive, maybe they're healthier. It's hard to know whether they show a benefit because of the amount of practice."

Dr. Greenberg noted that one of his studies examined the relationship between the amount of time people practiced yoga and the benefit they experienced.

"In that study, people were randomized to practice 40 minutes a day compared to either 10 minutes a day or between 10 minutes and 40 minutes a day. Only the group that was prescribed 40 minutes showed significantly reduced stress. That's why programs like Mindfulness-Based Stress Reduction and Mindfulness-Based Cognitive Therapy typically prescribe 40 minutes a day. That's something I would really try to adhere to. And even if you don't manage to make it the full 40 minutes— because some days you're not going to practice at all and maybe other nights you practice for 20—setting an intent to practice 40 minutes a day is beneficial. When trying to implement a regular practice, it is important to balance diligence with an attitude of compassion and kindness so that you're not too hard on yourself if you don't meet that standard. Most people don't reach 40 minutes a day, but setting the intention and striving toward it can be helpful."

Mindfulness is often used by athletes, actors, and performers who want to enhance their focus during moments of high stress. How can mindfulness be immediately helpful in such situations?

"Athletes, actors, and performers often face stress and sometimes anxiety toward a performance. Anxiety is, by definition, looking for an oncoming threat. Anxiety lies in the future. It says, 'Okay, something bad can happen, and I really need to be tuned toward what can possibly happen. . . . How can this go wrong, how can I respond to it?'

"Distractions often also come from dwelling on the past. A performer or athlete may ask themselves: 'Why did I miss that kick? Why did they not give me that part? I shouldn't have done this. I should have performed better.' This type of ruminative thinking has also been shown to be a risk factor for depression.

"We carry this baggage around . . . the baggage of our failures, the baggage of criticism, the baggage of our past experiences—if we're able to just set that aside and take that load off our shoulders, we're better able to see the freshness and newness of each event, each moment. So there's a great window of opportunity there to make things different if we focus on the task at hand and unload the baggage for a little bit."

In what settings is mindfulness taught?

"Mindfulness is being taught in settings like hospitals, primary care clinics, schools, prisons, and large corporations. Google has its own mindfulness teacher. It's being recognized that even having people spend 20 to 30 minutes a day meditating during work can increase productivity. To a limited degree, mindfulness is being gradually incorporated into military settings as well. . . . Most people who get drafted to the military will probably not encounter mindfulness training. But the growing body of research is having an effect, and we are seeing mindfulness training opportunities in a growing number of contexts."

ADDITIONAL STRESS MANAGEMENT TOOLS

Dr. Greenberg's insights and guidance provide us with a deeper understanding of how we might use mindfulness to manage stress, enhance our emotional and cognitive functioning, and boost our well-being. In addition to mindfulness, the following factors have been associated with decreased stress and enhanced well-being and cognitive functioning:

- *Spiritual fitness,* the study of how spirituality and/or religion help people cope with life's difficulties and experience greater joy, is an increasing area of study in the field of cognitive health and aging. In a recent review of 17 studies, 82 percent showed a positive link between spirituality and/or religion and cognitive functioning. It was concluded that spirituality and/or religion is protective against cognitive decline.[205]

- *Flow.* Dr. Mihaly Csikszentmihalyi, a prisoner during World War II who later became a happiness researcher, popularized the concept of flow. *Flow* is a state of optimal performance and engagement in tasks and activities that is characterized by enhanced attention (complete concentration and absorption in a task), a natural balance between skills and the challenge of the task, a sense of intrinsic reward, and "transformation of time" (a sense that time is moving faster or slower). Increased engagement in tasks and activities that are associated with flow is connected to greater feelings of well-being and happiness.

- *Resilience* is the ability to successfully adapt to stress, adversity, and trauma.[206] Several factors have been shown to promote resilience, including genetic factors that regulate responses to anxiety and stress, optimism, cognitive reframing (managing emotions by changing the way we think about an issue), identifying positive aspects of stressful events, "active coping" (changing the stressor and/or how it is perceived), social support, humor, exercise, altruism, and mindfulness.[207] Resilience also has been linked to spirituality.[208] Mastery of negative situations sometimes can inoculate a person against later stressors.

- **Positive stress management strategies.** You may already use several strategies to reduce your stress in "positive" ways (i.e., with methods that are generally not associated with long-term negative consequences). These might include the strategies noted above or common techniques such as the following:

- *Keeping a manageable schedule*

- *Preserving time with family and friends*

- *Removing yourself from stressful situations*

- *Reframing* (thinking about stressful situations differently)

- *Engaging in hobbies or relaxing activities* (taking walks, listening to music, taking a bath, journaling), doing deep breathing, and focusing on what we are grateful for in our lives

In contrast, negative, or nonadaptive, stress management strategies are behaviors that may help decrease stress in the short term but often have long-term negative consequences. These include smoking, drug use, excessive sleeping, emotional eating, and expressing emotions in ways that negatively affect relationships.

HIGH-OCTANE BRAIN ACTION PLAN: LOWER STRESS AND BOOST WELL-BEING

Reducing stress and enhancing mood and well-being are important to developing a High-Octane Brain. Let's put some stress management techniques to work for you.

💭 Reflect: Positive Stress Management

Identify three positive stress management tools you already use and jot them down in the "Positive Stress Management Tools" section under the "Chapter 7" heading of your High-Octane Action Plan. If you don't have positive stress management tools, write down three that you learned about in this chapter (or that you otherwise know about) that you'd like to try.

💭 Reflect: Recognize Your Resilience

Think about a challenging situation you experienced in which you exhibited resilience, the ability to thrive in the midst of stress and adversity. Write that situation down in the "Resilience in Action" section under the "Chapter 7" heading of your High-Octane Action Plan. Reminding yourself of your previous resilience sometimes helps you better navigate current stressful and challenging situations.

Next steps: If you would like to leverage the synergistic High-Octane Brain benefits of mindfulness, you can begin to learn more about it from the books and apps that were mentioned by Dr. Greenberg. A more personalized method for incorporating mindfulness into your daily life can be gained by participating in a mindfulness class.

> **"THE GREATEST WEAPON AGAINST STRESS IS OUR ABILITY TO CHOOSE ONE THOUGHT OVER ANOTHER."**
>
> —WILLIAM JAMES

📈 **Track:** This week, a fourth column has been added to the High-Octane Tracker to track your weekly stress level. This is the only step tracked on a weekly (versus daily) basis. At the end of the week, complete the "Lower Stress and Boost Well-Being" questions on the scoring page after the High-Octane Tracker (on pages 226 and 229). Then shade in the octane level for the total score on the brain diagram. Note that this column is "reverse scored," meaning that higher scores are associated with lower octane levels (fill up the octane levels from the bottom of the column on the diagram, just as you always do).

MEREDITH AND LOU: ADJUSTING AS THEY GO

Lou smiled as he held up his High-Octane Tracker. "My MIND diet score has already gone up a couple of points," he said. "I was in the 'Better' range last week for the first time."

Lou noticed that adding just two more healthy meals the week before made a big difference in his score. Al and Rachel had made him a chicken pasta casserole with spinach. "And I didn't even notice the spinach," he said, laughing.

Lou also reported that his mood was a bit happier, though he wasn't sure why. Many people find that they unexpectedly feel happier after improving their exercise, diet, and engagement. This synergistic effect often accelerates as the last two steps are added.

Meredith also brought in her High-Octane Tracker. Her "*Exercise*" was at the "Best" octane level, "*Consume Healthy Foods*" was at the "Better" level, and "*Engage*" was at the "Best" level. "So far, so good," she said, leaning forward but also looking a bit worried.

"I guess more than anything this week's class made me think about how I don't even have time for stress management," she explained. "I'd like to do mindfulness, but I don't have the time for that. And that makes me feel horrible, because I don't feel right not taking advantage of a technique that's so helpful to so many other areas."

I recommended that Meredith think back to what led her to want to improve her brain health in the first place. She'd been continuing to envision her Ideal Future Self when brushing her teeth and in many situations in which she was facing a Three-Path Choice. She noticed that her vision of herself in her garden was becoming more detailed and that she was feeling more joyful when she envisioned it. She also noticed that her Whys were evolving. This is very common as people start to engage in healthier habits and unexpected benefits—and goals—start to emerge.

Meredith shared her current Why: "To have better memory for myself. And not just out of fear . . . but so I can do all the things in the coming years that I don't even know I want to do yet . . . and do them really well."

This new Why seemed especially powerful for her, and realizing that made her more energized to make time for stress management. She was especially happy to hear that many people feel more productive when they improve their stress management. She admitted that she wanted to see an immediate impact from brain-healthy habits and was motivated to try mindfulness because of its amplified benefits (see page 134).

Both Meredith and Lou's experiences were typical of the High-Octane Brain approach. The more you love what you envision when you see your Ideal Future Self, the more powerful your Whys become and the more they will have the power to keep you on track in the midst of work, life, and all the other things that sometimes conspire to make brain health feel like it's not a priority.

TOP TAKEAWAYS

1. Chronic stress increases the risk of Alzheimer's, depression, and cardiovascular disease, among other health problems.

2. Mood and cognitive functioning are strongly connected: treatment of depression can enhance cognitive functioning, and happiness is linked to stronger cognitive performance.

3. Mindfulness—or "moment-to-moment nonjudgmental awareness"—is a highly effective stress management tool.

4. Spiritual fitness, flow, resilience, and positive stress management strategies also help decrease stress and boost well-being.

5. Amplified benefits occur when one step in the EXCELS Method positively impacts multiple other steps. Physical exercise and mindfulness provide the strongest amplified benefits in the EXCELS Method.

6. Identifying personal positive stress management strategies and examples of resilience in your High-Octane Action Plan can empower you to manage future stress more effectively.

CHAPTER 8

Step 5: **S**leep for Better Brain Power

"Sleep is the golden chain that ties health and our bodies together."

—THOMAS DEKKER

Although sleep researchers are constantly learning more about why we need sleep, one thing has been clear since the beginning of time: if we don't get enough of it, we falter.

Some of us have personally experienced the agony of sleep deprivation when taking care of a newborn baby, doing shift work, driving for long periods, or trying to meet a looming deadline. The effects of sleep deprivation may be subtle at first: our thinking may be a bit more sluggish, our memory not quite as precise, and our movements a bit slower. However, the impact tends to accelerate, and before we know it, we may feel like we are moving through the world in a slow-motion state of clumsiness and increasing confusion.

What is less obvious is that sleep deprivation actually impairs our ability to process and store the memories that we form during our waking hours. Further, if sleep deprivation is chronic (occurring over months or years), it may be a risk factor for Alzheimer's disease.

HOW TIRED ARE YOU?

Count the number of *A*'s in the following string of letters as quickly as you can:

F D S I B A F D K A A W E B W P E I J A G
E O P W D A B W E G E Q A P P E G H A

Now look around your environment and count how many red objects you see as quickly as you can.

Your speed and accuracy on these tasks (there were seven *A*'s above) is likely related at least partially to your answer to the following question:

How would you rate the quality of your sleep last night?

(**1** = very poor, **2** = poor, **3** = fair, **4** = good, **5** = very good)

People who rate their sleep quality as "poor" or "very poor" perform consistently lower on tasks that measure attention and speed of information processing. The impact of attention problems is wide-ranging and sometimes dangerous, contributing to deadly industrial accidents, medical mistakes, and 20 percent of traffic fatalities. In addition to poor sleep quality, about 40 percent of adults report that they do not get enough sleep.[209] That number may be an underestimate since people are notoriously inaccurate in determining whether they are well rested and often report that they are when their performance on tests suggests that they are not. In fact, their inaccuracy in perception may be related to poor sleep.

Sleep deprivation can compromise multiple stages of memory processing, including the ability to initially pay attention to and learn information and the ability to package and store that information once it has been learned. Furthermore, chronic sleep deprivation may increase the risk of Alzheimer's. Before we review the important links between sleep and memory, let's take a look at the different stages of sleep and why each stage is so important.

STAGES OF SLEEP

Sleep is broadly divided into two main categories: non-REM (rapid eye movement) sleep (stages 1–3) and REM sleep, as defined below:

Stage 1: Non-REM sleep: This initial stage of sleep, lasting several minutes, is characterized by a slowing of brain waves (alpha and theta waves), eye movements, heart rate, and breathing. People can generally be awakened easily at this stage.

Stage 2: Non-REM sleep: This stage is also only minutes long and is characterized by sudden increases in brain wave frequencies called sleep spindles.

Stage 3: Non-REM sleep: (slow-wave sleep [SWS]): This stage is associated with "restorative" sleep and contributes to the feeling of being refreshed. The brain starts to produce slow delta waves. Eye movement, heart rate, and breathing are at their lowest levels. This stage is associated with bodily tissue repair and growth and enhanced immune function.

Rapid eye movement: REM occurs about 90 minutes after a person falls asleep and usually lasts up to an hour. Most adults have five to six REM sleep episodes per night. This stage is where most dreaming occurs, eyes may move side to side, and breathing is rapid and irregular. REM periods lengthen throughout the night; that is why a dream may occur directly before awakening. The time we spend in REM sleep decreases as we age.

SLEEP AND MEMORY PROCESSING

There is much support for the role of SWS in selecting and packaging (consolidating) declarative memories and factual information (e.g., names of cities, people). The role of REM sleep in memory is less clear. Whereas some research has found that REM sleep is important for processing procedural memories (remembering *how* to do specific actions such as throwing a ball, walking, and knitting), other research suggests that SWS may be more important for packaging and storing procedural memories[210] and that REM may be more important for consolidation of emotional memories.[211]

There is also some evidence that both stages work together sequentially[212] so that specific memories may be selected and reactivated during SWS and that REM may help store those memories.[213] Recent research also suggests that the hippocampus plays a role in consolidating new memories even if it was not involved in learning the information initially.[214] Although many questions remain about the exact function of the sleep stages in memory processing, we *do* know that good sleep is vital to good memory.

SLEEP, COGNITIVE FUNCTIONING, AND ALZHEIMER'S DISEASE

Cross-cultural studies have provided additional support for the relationship between poor-quality sleep and cognitive symptoms.[215] Some research has shown that shorter and longer than average sleep durations are especially linked to cognitive impairment. For example, in an analysis of over 97,000 adults across 35 studies, those who slept less than five hours were 1.4 times more likely to have poorer memory, working memory (the ability to temporarily hold information in mind while completing a larger goal), and executive functions (strategy and judgment skills).[216] Those who slept more than nine hours per night were 1.58 times more likely to have such issues.[217] A recent study supported this finding, showing that in 1,500 adults age 60 or older, those who slept 10 hours or more had poorer performance on tasks of memory, rapid verbal expression, processing speed, and working memory.[218] Other studies have shown a relationship between sleep duration, sleep fragmentation, and sleep-disordered breathing and later dementia,[219] with one study estimating that individuals with sleep problems have a 1.68 times higher risk of Alzheimer's and that about 15 percent of cases of Alzheimer's may be related to sleep problems.[220] These findings have fueled a growing interest in studying sleep to lower the risk of Alzheimer's.[221]

 Individuals with sleep problems have lower cognitive functioning and a higher rate of Alzheimer's.

Dr. Brendan Lucey on Sleep, Cognitive Functioning, and Alzheimer's

Brendan Lucey, MD, is the director of sleep medicine and assistant professor of neurology at Washington University School of Medicine. His research on the relationship between sleep deprivation and increased levels of beta-amyloid and tau—proteins involved in Alzheimer's—has received widespread recognition for its importance.

Why is sleep so important to cognitive functioning?

"There are several different ways that sleep disturbances can impact cognitive function. The very basic way is simply through lack of attention. If someone is sleep-deprived, he or she is not going to be able to attend as well to whatever he or she is doing or attempting to learn. For instance, if a sleep-deprived individual is reading, he or she may not able to capture the information the same way."

How might sleep deprivation relate to Alzheimer's?

"There's a lot of evidence that we and others have showing that sleep changes with Alzheimer's disease pathology. The field is simultaneously pursuing two different but related hypotheses. There's a proposed bidirectional relationship in Alzheimer's disease. . . . The pathology of Alzheimer's disease disrupts sleep, and sleep disruption promotes Alzheimer's pathology in the other direction, going back and forth. Once one of these starts off, it creates this feedback loop that accelerates the process."

What types of Alzheimer's-related cellular abnormalities are linked to sleep deprivation?

"A lot of work we've been doing at Washington University is taking findings from mouse models and trying to translate them to humans. In mice, we know that amyloid beta [a protein involved in Alzheimer's] goes up and down with the sleep-wake cycle. That was then shown to be true in humans as well. My lab had a paper last year (2018) where cognitively normal participants 30 to 60 years old were sleep deprived and given a drug to help them sleep or allowed to sleep normally. We showed you can increase amyloid beta by about 30 percent with complete sleep deprivation. . . . Other studies showed that if someone 10 years earlier was complaining of daytime sleepiness, they're much more likely to develop amyloid pathology even if they're cognitively normal.

"The reason we think sleep loss could promote Alzheimer's disease pathology with amyloid deposition is that amyloid deposition is concentration-dependent. So the higher the concentration is, the more likely amyloid beta is to aggregate as plaque. If you don't drop your concentration overnight due to good sleep, it's going to stay persistently elevated. I don't think that a single night of sleep loss would be a problem, but 20 years of persistently elevated amyloid beta may start or accelerate the process of depositing amyloid as plaque.

"In collaboration with Dave Holtzman's lab here at Washington University—who had first described the oscillation of amyloid beta with sleep-wake activity in mice and showed that tau also changes with sleep-wake activity—we went back to samples of the fluid around the brain that I collected [in humans] and also showed that tau increases with sleep deprivation. The reason that's potentially important is that there's a hypothesis about 'tau spreading': in synaptically linked neural networks, once tau starts to accumulate in neurons, it can spread out to other neighboring neurons. They [Dr. Holtzman's lab] were able to show in mice that sleep loss increased the spreading of tau. We obviously couldn't show that in humans, but we did show that sleep loss increased the amount of tau, raising the potential at least that this could be a mechanism for tau spreading.

"Amyloid deposition precedes the onset of cognitive symptoms by 15 to 20 years. Amyloid deposition in itself isn't sufficient to develop Alzheimer's disease. You have to have the amyloid deposition and then the tau pathology, which is about five to seven years before symptom onset. Tau is what really causes the problem, because intracellular tau leads to neuronal and synaptic loss and you lose enough neurons that your memory starts to become affected. There's a long lead time."

Why is there such a large focus on the role of slow-wave sleep and Alzheimer's?

"Slow-wave activity is a measure of sleep quality. It's part of the homeostatic sleep drive. So as you're awake, you develop an increased need to sleep. Combined with your circadian rhythm, or internal clock, that helps promote sleep at night. So when you go to sleep, your slow-wave activity is very high early in the night. As you pay off your 'sleep debt,' or sleep need, your slow-wave activity decreases and you don't have as much slow-wave activity as the night goes on. We looked at the average of all-night slow-wave activity. Those who had lower slow-wave activity had increased amyloid and tau on brain scans. If you think about slow-wave activity as the restorative quality of sleep, it's impaired.

"Slow-wave activity decreases with age, [and there are] significant sex differences in slow-wave activity in older adults. Women as they get older lose much less slow-wave sleep than men. Slow-wave sleep when you're younger is approximately 18 percent of the night; older women drop down to about 10 to 12 percent, whereas men [drop down to] less than about 5 percent. One prediction would be that women are protected from getting Alzheimer's disease; however, women are actually at increased risk of Alzheimer's disease. . . . Clearly the relationship between sleep and Alzheimer's disease is complex."

How might the study of sleep potentially inform treatments for Alzheimer's?

"Long before I started doing research on Alzheimer's disease, there was a big push to characterize the preclinical phase of disease, when there is evidence of Alzheimer's pathology but no cognitive problems with thinking and memory. The Alzheimer's disease pathology is defined by the biomarkers for amyloid and tau in the brain. The idea is that interventions for Alzheimer's disease may be failing because we are treating symptomatic people, and if you can push back the time when you're going to be doing the intervention . . . even before they develop symptoms, it's more likely to be helpful. The idea being that once those neurons are dying . . . you're not going to bring those neurons back."

How is the relationship between sleep and Alzheimer's studied?
"In looking at sleep disturbances causing Alzheimer's pathology, a lot of work is done in two big groups of studies: one is bench research like in animal models or studies with a small number of humans—small clinical translational projects. And there are other studies using large cohorts of participants that measured sleep in some way—objective measures like a sleep study or a questionnaire—and then they were followed for cognitive outcomes or amyloid PET [positron emission tomography] scans."

How much sleep is optimal?
"Most people need seven to eight hours of sleep. And just simply budgeting that time is lacking for a lot of individuals, myself included. Although some people don't need as much sleep, the majority do, and most people underestimate the amount of sleep they need."

How can people improve sleep quality?
"Most people could focus on sleep hygiene issues like keeping a regular routine and getting up and reading in low light before returning to bed if they are having problems falling asleep." Dr. Lucey also explained that Cognitive Behavioral Therapy for Insomnia (CBTI) can also be very helpful in treating insomnia and that it is crucial to treat any sleep disorders. For example, sleep apnea (a condition in which breathing repeatedly stops and starts during sleep) may require treatment with

CPAP (continuous positive airway pressure) therapy. He noted that future research may focus on how to increase compliance with CPAP therapy in older adults and develop related protocols.

What are the biggest challenges in improving sleep?

"American society as a whole is really chronically sleep deprived. And there are really good data over the last 20 years showing that we're not very good at perceiving how impaired we are from chronic sleep deprivation. There's a number of things that can go on when you have chronic poor sleep. Your performance can deteriorate, but also how much you appreciate that performance decline can change. You may not realize that you're as impaired as you actually are.

"There's a very interesting study from about 20 years ago that equated sleep deprivation and alcohol content in the blood with reaction time performance. It's like you're legally drunk when you've been awake for 24 to 30 hours. If you think about impairments, most people will understand how alcohol can impair your judgment and thinking. Equating it to that is a helpful thing to point out to people.

"With some older adults, they are sent in by their primary care doctor for sleep apnea, and they often equate it to getting older, so they think they're supposed to sleep terribly. And then we treat their sleep disorder, they realize, 'I'm not supposed to sleep terribly.' And their sleep is much improved. There is an implicit bias that we all have that as we get older, we have a lot more medical problems."

What are the challenges in researching sleep and Alzheimer's?

"I think this line of research looking at the relationships between sleep and Alzheimer's disease in older adults shows a lot of promise in looking for it as a marker of Alzheimer's disease or an intervention to prevent or delay it, but . . . in some ways the complexity is going to increase simply because the causes of sleep disturbance in older adults are many."

What led to your interest in researching sleep and Alzheimer's?
"Five years ago, there was a lot of interesting research on sleep in animal models and beginning data in humans as well. It was an exciting area with discoveries to be made. It's also a very important field. In neurology, there are few areas that are as much of a public health crisis as Alzheimer's."

Sleep: Best Practices

1. *Adequate sleep is critical to cognitive functioning.* Most adults need seven to eight hours of sleep.

2. *It is important to recognize and treat existing sleep problems.* It is important to seek medical attention to treat any sleep-related problems. Sleep apnea affects about 9 to 38 percent of adults (with rates in older adults as high as 90 percent in men and 78 percent in women).[222] In addition, about 30 percent of the world population reports symptoms of insomnia, including difficulty falling asleep, staying asleep, and getting back to sleep and poor sleep quality.[223] The following treatments have been shown to be beneficial for individuals with insomnia:

   A. *Cognitive Behavioral Treatment for Insomnia (CBTI).* This treatment is highly effective, though access to it may be limited.[224]

   B. *"Sleep hygiene"* (behavioral strategies to enhance sleep), as explained in the section on pages 160–62.

   C. *Physical exercise,*[225] including aquatic exercise,[226] and even a single session of light-intensity walking.[227] In addition, a combination of aerobic exercise and sleep hygiene techniques is linked to improved sleep quality, mood, and quality of life.[228]

D. *Mindfulness.* A recent randomized controlled trial showed that mindfulness was as successful as CBTI and sleep medication in treating moderate sleep disturbances in older adults in a community-accessible model. The therapeutic impact of mindfulness was attributed to the ability to decrease activation of the autonomic nervous system (heart rate, breathing) through a learned relaxation response. Mindfulness also decreased sleep-related daytime impairment, potentially enhancing the quality of life.[229]

E. *Volunteering* has been associated with improvements in sleep, possibly as a result of increased physical, cognitive, and social activity,[230] though it has not been studied as widely.

F. *Sleep medications.* Although sleep medications are widely used, the sedative effects of some medications can compromise the restorative benefits of sleep. In addition, approximately 80 percent of older adults report at least one side effect from sleep medication (typically drowsiness, difficulty concentrating, or impaired memory) that interferes with functioning at home, at work, and in social relationships.[231]

BOOST YOUR SLEEP QUALITY

Behavioral and environmental strategies (sleep hygiene techniques) are an effective treatment for many individuals with insomnia.[232]

Here are some recommended strategies:

- *Get out of bed and do something relaxing if you can't fall asleep after 10 to 15 minutes.* Relaxing activities might include reading under low light and listening to soft music (but not tasks that increase alertness, such as doing the dishes). Then return to bed when you feel tired. It may seem counterintuitive to get out of bed, but staying in bed and trying to fall asleep can compromise future sleep by teaching your brain to link lying in bed with *not* falling asleep. Over time, engaging in a relaxing activity before returning to bed often leads people to fall asleep faster.

- *Create a relaxing bedtime nighttime ritual.* The brain quickly learns to associate actions that occur in sequence. By following a relaxing ritual—perhaps by shutting off electronic devices, turning down the lights, and spending time reading or taking a warm bath—you can teach your brain to move into a more relaxed mode the next time you start your bedtime routine. Over time, this can help your brain anticipate sleep and help you fall asleep faster.

- **Minimize blue light exposure.** Blue light from televisions, laptops, smartphones, and other electronic devices can interfere with the body's sleep-wake cycle. Turning off devices about one hour before bed and/or using a blue light filter can help minimize these effects. One study showed that blocking blue light improved working memory and the speed of information processing in individuals with insomnia.[233]

- *Follow a regular sleep schedule.* It's important to go to bed and wake up around the same time every day, even on weekends. Try not to nap, as naps often disrupt the sleep schedule.

- *Create a sleep haven.* Make sure your bedroom is cool, dark, and quiet. Ensure that your mattress and pillows are comfortable.

- *Exercise.* Exercise is linked with falling asleep faster and sleeping more soundly as long as you don't exercise less than one hour before bed.

- *Limit caffeine.* Try not to use it for at least six hours before bed.[234]

- *Limit alcohol.* Try not to drink it for at least three hours before bed. Although alcohol at bedtime is linked to falling asleep faster, it leads to lighter sleep and more awakenings after it is metabolized during the first few hours of sleep.[235] (It also is associated with increased alpha waves from stage 1 that disrupt slow-wave sleep.)

THE SYNERGY OF SLEEP

As we've discussed in previous chapters, one of the greatest benefits of the EXCELS Method is its synergistic effects. A positive feedback loop is created as brain health habits are added together. They begin to promote one another, and by doing so, brain health improves and creates an increased ability to continue using the habits. Sleep provides one of the most powerful synergistic effects. For example, enhanced sleep improves energy, which is associated with greater engagement in physical and cognitive activities and lower stress levels. Treatment of insomnia is also associated with decreased depression[236] and increased well-being. Good sleep also contributes to an increased emotional buffer, possibly because it provides enhanced cognitive ability to put things into perspective and weigh multiple factors.

HIGH-OCTANE BRAIN ACTION PLAN: SLEEP FOR BETTER BRAIN POWER

 Reflect: Improving Your Sleep

Review the "Boost Your Sleep Quality" feature on the previous page. Write down three sleep tips you think would be most helpful in enhancing your sleep quality in the "Top Actions to Improve Sleep" section under the "Chapter 8" heading of your High-Octane Action Plan. Try to integrate at least one of those tips consistently over the next week. Add a new tip only after you have incorporated the previous tip successfully for a full week.

Track: Monitor your daily sleep quality every morning by completing the sleep-quality question on the scoring page in your High-Octane Tracker (see page 230). At the end of the week, average your sleep quality score and fill in the octane level corresponding with that number on the front of the brain diagram. This is the last of the five steps to track in the EXCELS Method.

MEREDITH AND LOU: CHANGES TAKE HOLD

Lou looked as if a weight had been lifted from him. "I have sleep apnea. . . . I guess I stop breathing a lot at night, and that cuts off the oxygen to my brain. I was really worried, but the doctor said it's pretty common. She said I can wear a sleeping mask to help. She also said something about it maybe being connected to my depression."

Treating sleep apnea can help with other commonly related issues, including problems with attention and memory and depression. Lou continued to notice an improvement in his mood and was looking forward to seeing whether treatment of his sleep apnea would boost his mood even further.

Meredith recounted that she had spent 10 to 15 minutes a day the previous week practicing mindfulness. She noticed that she was sleeping better and wasn't sure if it was because of mindfulness, exercise, or just because she was feeling better overall. But she was concerned about the research showing Alzheimer's-related cellular changes after just one night of sleep deprivation. However, she was comforted to learn that researchers believe that chronic sleep deprivation over a period of years is the most concerning issue.

Lou then asked how she'd been able to carve out time for mindfulness given her concerns the week before. Meredith explained that she asked her husband to help with some of the rides for their grandchildren and enlisted her colleagues to help with a project at work.

"I can't say I put myself first, but I'm a little higher on the list than I was," she said. "It seems so obvious now, but I guess I didn't realize before that my brain is the common denominator of everything in my life, so if it isn't in tip-top shape, then nothing that I do with it can be either."

Because the next week of tracking would be the last step in the EXCELS Method (*Sleep*), we took time to reflect on Meredith and Lou's progress since starting the program.

Meredith began by recalling her initial fear about Alzheimer's: "I'm still terrified of it, to tell you the truth. I don't know if that will ever go away. But what's different is that now I feel like I'm doing all I can to either stop it from happening or delay when it does happen. And that makes me feel much better than just being scared."

Lou said his biggest change was feeling more motivated to improve his brain health and mood. He recalled how he initially agreed to the program because he promised his son he would. "But now I'm doing it because it makes me feel good," he admitted. "And actually kind of 'blah' if I don't. . . . I didn't expect that."

We wrapped up the session by discussing the importance of continuing to envision the connection between their Ideal Future Self and the Three-Path Choice, to connect with their evolving Whys, and to remember that the OCTANE acronym (*One Change at a Time Accomplished Now equals Excellence*) at the top of the High-Octane Tracker was there to remind them that any positive change—no matter how small—was a sign of progress.

TOP TAKEAWAYS

1. The average adult needs seven or eight hours of sleep. Sleeping less than five hours or more than nine hours a night is linked to higher rates of cognitive impairment.

2. Poor sleep impairs attention and memory and is linked to a higher rate of Alzheimer's.

3. Sleep hygiene techniques are very effective in enhancing sleep quality (see pages 160–62).

4. There are four stages of sleep, each with characteristic brain waves and functions. Slow-wave sleep (stage 3) helps process and store factual information. REM sleep helps process and store emotions and memory of how to carry out specific physical actions.

5. You can enhance your sleep quality by choosing tailored strategies to address specific sleep problems (see pages 159–60) and by tracking your sleep quality.

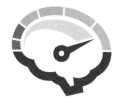

PART III

High-Octane Brain
Role Models

"The big question is whether you are going to be able to say a hearty yes to your adventure."

—Joseph Campbell

CHAPTER 9

Meet Your Brain Health Success Squad: High-Octane Brain Role Models Ages 44 to 83

"But do you know how old I will be by the time I learn to really play the piano / act / paint / write a decent play?"
"Yes . . . the same age you will be if you don't."

—JULIA CAMERON

This chapter includes profiles of five High-Octane Brain role models who range in age from 44 to 83 years.* Chapter 10 includes four profiles of High-Octane Brain role models between ages 91 and 103. Each of the role models reported engaging in high levels of brain healthy habits across most of the five steps in the EXCELS Method. Their stories are presented to highlight the success that is possible on the journey of the High-Octane Brain even in the context of significant life challenges and stress.

The content of each interview was captured through broad, open-ended questions to allow the role models to self-identify the aspects of their life stories that they felt were most important. This made the overlapping themes that emerged even more meaningful.

The stories of these role models are presented to help us see the journey of brain health in expanded ways and to open up new ideas for exploration as our own brain health journeys unfold. I hope you're as inspired by them as I was. Each time I reviewed them, another unique facet stood out, beckoning me to see the life stories—and imagine the possibilities of our collective stories—from new angles.

Reflect: Who and What Inspires You?

As you read the stories of the High-Octane Brain role models in this chapter and the next, write down the themes and role models that speak to you. Then, in the "Top Insights" section under the "Chapters 9 and 10" heading of your High-Octane Action Plan on page 218, write down your top three (or more) insights.

*NOTE: Ages given for each role model reflect their age at the time of their interviews.

Amy

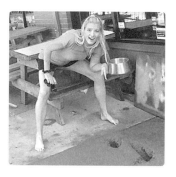

AGE: 44 (birth date 1974)
BIRTHPLACE: Traverse County, Minnesota
OCCUPATION: Geropsychologist

The youngest of eight children, Amy recalled that being raised on a farm in western Minnesota with her "hands in the dirt" and "fresh organic food" deeply shaped her lifestyle and habits. These days she loves picking berries, making smoothies, and spending time outdoors in the Pacific Northwest with her partner, Jeff, and their three-year-old daughter and one-year-old son. She especially loves to model healthy eating for her children and show them how she checks off a calendar to track foods on the MIND diet. "It makes me really happy to be able to give them that," she told me, laughing, "even though it's not something I'm actually physically handing to them."

Amy recalled that her father's work as an entrepreneur and her "familial work ethic to be productive" instilled in her an expectation that she would do well in school and be successful. "I was going to do well," she explained. "It was a belief system." It fed her desire to attend graduate school, where she studied geropsychology and combined her love of science with her desire to help older adults live with passion and thrive in the context of challenge.

"One Breath at a Time"

During her times of challenge and especially in the midst of loss, Amy has found comfort by focusing on "one breath at a time." She recalled that the death of her beloved father last year, the day before the birth of her son, was something for which she only recently "took the time to grieve." She also reflected on another profound challenge, when her life was upended a few years ago after she ended her marriage. "In the throes of those events," she said, "there's this sense of 'How in the world can you possibly continue on?'" She found solace in "identifying with the parts of life that didn't appear to be ending." Amy added: "My life was not just one thing or relationship or set of difficult circumstances . . . there were so many different dimensions, and most of them were vibrant, moving, and filled with energy in some way."

"I did not fall over and die at any of those points," she explained. "I sometimes felt like I should have, but I didn't. When I thought there was no way I could make it through something like this . . . there I was standing on the other side, a better person." Amy believed that spirituality, mindfulness, writing, and connecting with nature and the "essence of energy" from others in a "visceral way" also played a "very big role" in grounding her.

Amy feels that her healthy lifestyle has become somewhat automatic and was set in motion through a combination of exposure and mind-set, especially in regard to exercise. She recalled that in childhood, "My surroundings encouraged me to feel athletic," and led her to make exercise a habit. She continues to prioritize exercise in the midst of raising her young family and attending to her professional obligations by asking herself, "'What really matters to me? What is it that if I haven't done it, I feel some sense of dissatisfaction or unhappiness?'" To Amy, exercise became a clear example of something that was simply part of what she did. "I don't have to make myself exercise anymore," she said. "Because it's such a habit that I feel yucky if I don't do it."

A New Trajectory

Since starting a family in her forties, Amy has experienced a profound and unexpected shift in the trajectory of her life plan. "Balancing children and work with a very young family" has led her to feel that "instead of continuing on in the chronological age trajectory where I was or where I'm at in terms of my actual numerical age, it feels like I basically rewound time 10 to 15 years." She added that her decision to start a family blossomed from a desire to create "close emotional bonds" and "intimate relationships," which have led to a life she cherishes. Her current life, she feels, is partly born from her resilience. "The blossoming seed that came from the challenging times is the best thing that I could imagine," she said. "Those experiences have made me a better person."

> *"This new trajectory . . . it just seemed to happen by doing things I thought would be healthy and wonderful."*

In accordance with her new trajectory, Amy looks forward to working into her nineties, whether in the world of psychology or with one of the creative endeavors she often dreams up but doesn't have time to pursue. In the meantime, one of her more pressing realities is interrupted sleep, especially since the birth of her son last year. "It's so disrupted, I don't even know how to count it," she explained, laughing. "If I at least get six and a half hours, I can function. And then seven or eight is just dreamy. If I have eight hours where my head is kind of close to the pillow most of the time, that is spectacular."

Health History

Family medical history: Some of Amy's family members have had memory problems.

Medical history: Amy does not have any major health issues and does not smoke.

Brain Health Highlights

Memory function: Amy has exceptional memory for future tasks such as remembering to pick up specific items from the grocery store and uses strategies to remember them. She notices minor memory problems and word-finding difficulties (mostly when she is sleep deprived) but feels they are normal for her age.

Exercise: Amy exercises at least four times a week, for one hour per day, and enjoys a variety of activities, including cross-training, jogging, hiking, weight lifting, biking, yoga, basketball, and volleyball.

Activities and cognitive engagement: Amy enjoys reading and exploring local markets and festivals. She often tries to learn a new "word of the day" and seeks other opportunities to learn new information on a daily basis.

Diet: Amy and her family follow the MIND diet, which she tracks on a large calendar. She notes that her family is "berry-centric" and they often pick their own berries. She and her family do not eat fried food and have very few processed foods. Amy has one daily serving of "craft beer or awesome wine from the Pacific Northwest."

Sleep: Amy sleeps about six to seven hours per night, though currently her sleep is interrupted by caring for her young children.

Mood: Amy described her mood as "very happy."

Social engagement: Amy enjoys spending time with her family, friends, and neighbors.

Top brain health habit: Making a decision to engage in a healthy behavior. "It's the principle of once you've decided, you don't get to debate it anymore. Once you've made up your mind, you can let go of the mental dialogue."

Advice to others who wish to strengthen their brain health: "Follow your passion. It's only what you truly care about that will motivate you."

Virgil

AGE: 53 (birth date 1965)

BIRTHPLACE: Lake County, Illinois

OCCUPATION: Pharmaceutical sales

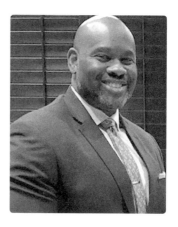

Raised on the south side of Chicago, Virgil recalled that his childhood was "pretty normal" until his parents divorced when he was 13 years old. After that, he and his mother and four siblings moved to the Chicago suburbs, where they endured many years of "serious poverty," with little water or food. "I used to drive my mother's car with a trash can and put water in it," he recalled. "That was our water to wash with. So we were living in the suburbs with our basic needs not really being met." Those experiences, he explained, "have led me to celebrate the little things a bit more than some folks do."

Lessons from the Football Field

After high school, Virgil noticed that exercise gave him something unexpectedly powerful: "I could control how my body looked, so I really jumped into exercise. And that was kind of my place to have some happiness."

That happiness propelled Virgil to pursue a goal he'd been told he would never achieve. He walked onto a legendary football field at Central State University, a small historically black school in Ohio, and tried out for the team. Not only did he win the starting free safety job, but it led to a scholarship. His success on the field also came with an unexpected discovery off it: the power of diet.

"I would clean my diet up as we got into the season," Virgil explained, "because I had to be able to study. A lot of guys would drink. Not me. During the season, I would keep it as clean as I could, because I found I could think better."

When something isn't going optimally for Virgil, he first examines his diet to see what changes need to be made. He found that adjusting diet and exercise "helps you think clearly and have your daily wins . . . your monthly, weekly wins, so that even though maybe work isn't going great, that particular part of your life can go pretty well."

Virgil enjoys sharing his insights with others who seek his guidance to improve their health. He draws from his previous work as a personal trainer with over 30 years of bodybuilding experience. He tries to get people to focus on what truly motivates them beyond their fitness goals. "What is your real goal?" he asks. "What is it that you want?"

Virgil stressed the need to have a plan: "So if my career goal is to be a manager in two years, then I have steps in place for that. The fitness, the diet, has to go into that." He encourages others to strengthen their brain health, specifically to "try to be the best version of yourself consistently." Doing that sets the stage for continuous learning, he explained.

> *"If you aren't learning something new at least every couple of days, you tend to fall back into something not as desirable."*

Always Reach Higher

Virgil is committed to continuous learning, which is something he encourages in others, too. He seeks fresh ways to enhance his exercise routines, reviewing research, videos, and new exercise apps. Virgil also tries to continuously improve his brain health: "I believe I have very good control over my brain health as long as I continue to research and continue to be open to new things." He isn't afraid to get input from others.

"I have the ability to say 'I'm not good at that,'" he said. "I need to read, research, and call someone or figure out how I can achieve that goal."

Virgil has enjoyed great success in pharmaceutical sales for the last 19 years despite his career trajectory taking a hit after he had to "restart the clock" at age 40 while raising two daughters and a son after a divorce. Now that his children are graduating from college, he plans to increase his focus on his career. In the next few years, he would like to become a pharmaceutical division manager. In the longer term, he may pursue his college dream of becoming a lawyer.

A final, crucial part of Virgil's success, he noted, is staying within yourself: "You need to know you will never have it all figured out."

Health History

Family medical history: Virgil has no family history of memory problems.
Medical history: Virgil has sleep apnea. He does not smoke. He had a couple of concussions while playing football in college.

Brain Health Highlights

Memory function: Virgil believes that maximizing his memory is very important. He has some difficulty recalling small details but feels that his memory is normal for his age.
Exercise: Virgil lifts weights four to six days per week for 75 minutes a day and does cardiovascular exercise two to three times per week for 30 minutes a day. For the last 10 years, he has done martial arts twice per week for 90 minutes a day.
Activities and cognitive engagement: Virgil enjoys fashion, volunteering, and learning new information about nutrition and exercise.
Diet: Virgil eats four to six meals per day, including a protein shake in the morning. He eats two servings of omega-3 fatty acids a day, at least four servings of whole grains, and at least four servings of dark green leafy vegetables. He eats more than four servings of berries a week and does not eat processed foods. He drinks alcohol three to four times per month.

Sleep: Virgil sleeps four to six hours per night and generally feels well rested.

Mood: He describes his mood as "extremely happy."

Social engagement: Virgil enjoys spending time with his two daughters and his son, other family members, friends, and colleagues.

Top brain health habit: Virgil believes that exercise strengthens his mental sharpness and overall success.

Advice to others who wish to strengthen their brain health: "Try to be the best version of yourself consistently."

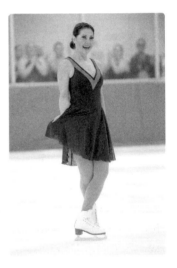

Jan

AGE: 62 (birth date 1957)

BIRTHPLACE: Sheboygan County, Wisconsin

OCCUPATION: Salon owner

As I watched Jan glide across the ice in May 2019, deftly completing swizzles and turns, I marveled at her grace and speed. She learned to figure skate at age 31, taking lessons with 5-year-olds while her 11-year-old daughter learned with her peers. Since picking up the sport again in her forties, she has competed in synchronized skating, free skating, and ice dancing. One of her proudest moments came at age 56, when she completed a complicated move that took her years to learn: the "death spiral." The move required her to arch backward on one foot as her body hovered just inches above the ice, circling her coach at high speeds as he held on to her with one hand. "You learn to be fearless," she said. "It's resilience . . . because we fall down so much in skating, it's like you've got to get back up because that's just a part of it . . . and it's a part of life."

Love and Tenacity

Jan recalled that her earliest lessons in perseverance came from her mother, who taught her that "you can choose to be better than your circumstances." Her mother, a Japanese orphan who worked in a factory as a child, was sent to Hiroshima at age 16 to care for victims of the atomic bomb. Jan recalled that though the victims were often gravely wounded and severely burned, her mother always tried to comfort and reassure them.

Jan's parents met in Tokyo, where her father was stationed during the Korean War. They later moved to the United States. Jan said that her mother "was always optimistic and lived her life with gratitude" in spite of experiencing racism while also raising Jan and her three siblings with limited resources after her divorce from Jan's father.

"Her attitude was always 'We might not have a lot, but we have love,'" Jan said. "If somebody was horrible to her, she would demonstrate how to be above that. I think that stemmed from knowing what it was like to be hurt, hungry, starving, or afraid. She decided, 'I will choose not to be that way.' No matter what happens in my life, no matter how horrible things are, I remember that example from my mom."

When her mother developed significant memory problems, Jan recalled, "I saw memory loss, but I also saw no effort at all to do anything to make good health choices with food or exercise." Instead, her mother would say, "Oh, well, I'm 78, or I'm 63. What do you expect?"

"I'm aware that it [memory problems] could be part of my genetic blueprint," Jan admitted. "I'm focusing on everything I can do to be healthy. I firmly believe the choices I make can help maybe slow down what might be inevitable genetically and that I have the control to enhance the quality of my life by remaining physically active. I'm continuing to move along a path of choosing good food . . . getting sleep . . . I'm not overthinking or worrying about it. I used to be worried about it, and now I just figure, 'Go with the flow.'"

"Maybe it will work, maybe it won't.
Who knows? Let's try."

New Frontiers

When Jan was 51, her 11-year-old son asked her to learn to snowboard with him. She remembers initially thinking, "I'm 51, I can't do that," and then realizing, "You could . . . you don't know." Just as she had done with figure skating, she first learned to snowboard by taking lessons with children. Even though she was "uncoordinated" and not athletic in childhood, she progressed quickly—partly because of the agility and balance she developed in figure skating—and was surprised by her success. She remembers thinking, "Who knew I could go into the terrain park at my age and do a boardslide off a rail?" She went on to become a snowboard instructor from ages 53 to 58. Just as figure skating set the stage for snowboarding, it prepared her for a variety of fitness activities she is currently involved in, including kickboxing, Zumba, and, most recently, bowling.

Jan's engagement in sports is inspired by healthy role models. Her 87-year-old former father-in-law, who is "mentally sharp and plays racquetball three times a week," often competing against men who are decades younger, has been particularly influential. "When I see people my age who are running marathons or coming here to the rink and skating," she said, "you see not just their physical fitness but their whole presence . . . those are people you pay attention to."

Jan feels her active lifestyle not only balances her job as a salon owner but has "connected me to people and contributed to my emotions, mental health, and well-being." Her social circle has been especially important to her since her divorce last year. "I had to learn how to be alone," she explained, noting how helpful it was to join Facebook groups, socialize with people in her fitness classes and at church, and start dating again. "I feel like despite all the things that have happened and all the different cycles in my life and transitions," she said, "I have a real sense of feeling grateful and feeling grounded."

Jan's next goal is to learn archery. "I'll think about being the age I feel," she explained. "I feel 36 years old. So my mind feels 36, and then it's like, 'Okay, body, let's go, because we're 36. We can do this and just have fun.'"

Health History

Family medical history: Jan's mother had undiagnosed memory problems and died at age 79. Her father died at age 72.

Medical history: Jan has no health problems and does not smoke.

Brain Health Highlights

Memory function: Jan experiences minor memory problems but feels they are common for her age.

Exercise: Jan ice skates four hours a week and does other cardiovascular exercise at least four days a week for 45 minutes at a time. She enjoys kickboxing, Zumba, snowboarding, and bowling and plans to learn archery. She was a snowboard instructor from ages 53 to 58.

Activities and cognitive engagement: Jan works full-time as a salon owner/manager and is active on Facebook. She also enjoys learning the cognitive components of a variety of sports.

Diet: Jan eats three to five servings of dark green leafy vegetables and four or more servings of berries per week, three or more servings of whole grains each day, and one serving of processed food per week. She does not drink alcohol.

Sleep: Jan sleeps seven or more hours a night and feels well rested most days.

Mood: She is "content" and happy most days.

Social engagement: Jan enjoys spending time with family and friends and dating.

Top brain health habit: "Remember that you can choose to be better than your circumstances."

Advice to others who wish to strengthen their brain health: "Remember what brought you joy when you were a kid and explore that. That's what I did with ice skating. I loved skating as a kid. I mean, we grew up really poor . . . but somehow my mom got us ice skates and skating was free, so I would go skating after school and on the weekends. I just enjoyed the wind against my face and the running around."

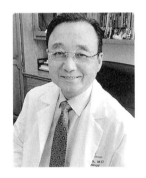

Byung

AGE: 72 (birth date 1946)

BIRTHPLACE: Gwangju, South Korea

OCCUPATION: Neurologist

At age 27, Byung, his wife, Jenny, and their baby, Erin, made the long voyage from Korea to Hawaii. Then they moved to Ohio, where Byung completed his medical internship and residency and they began to raise their children. Shortly after their arrival, prompted by Jenny's long-standing quest for the meaning of life, she encouraged Byung to attend church. "I was so ignorant of the spiritual world," Byung remembered. "I was a science guy throughout my schooling . . . so I opened my mind to learn more about the spiritual world." He didn't expect his newfound Christian faith to help guide him during the challenges that lay ahead.

After three years of medical training, Byung joined a thriving family practice in Illinois. But he quickly became dissatisfied with his lack of specialty training in caring for patients with neurological issues, including stroke, multiple sclerosis, and Parkinson's disease. He soon realized, "I don't think I want to stay as a generalist . . . this is not me. I'm too young to practice for 40 years like this."

Unexpected Fulfillment

After much deliberation and a belief that "God would provide a way," Byung made the decision to specialize in neurology. That required an additional three years of training, significant time away from his wife and two young children, and financial hardship as he shifted back to becoming a trainee. He recalled that the decision was particularly difficult because others "thought I was crazy" and told him, "You had a good practice opportunity, a partner, a good location . . . why do you want to go back to training for three more years?" He smiled, noting, "Jenny supported me with her whole heart, and so I was able to finish."

In early 2006, after several of his colleagues retired, Byung faced uncertainty about where he would continue his neurology practice. After declining offers to join various medical practices, he spearheaded a deal to ensure that he and 12 other staff members and colleagues, some of whom he had worked with for decades, would continue working together. "That was one of the best decisions I have made in my life," he said. "I was so happy, because everybody's happy." Byung smiled as he recalled that if he had not specialized in neurology years earlier, he would not have had the privilege of working with his beloved colleagues and "work family." "It was a divine appointment," he declared.

A Life-Changing Turning Point

In November 2018, Byung's wife of 46 years passed away after a several-year battle with cancer. "My better half is gone," he says sadly. "So I'm just functioning with the other half, which is not as good as the other part. That's how I feel. So when I think of that, I just have no desire to do anything." Byung is still struggling with the loss. "I cannot create new memories with my wife," he explained, offering a window into his thinking. "I only have past memories, which is very difficult to cope with." He said that working sometimes distracts from his loss, but "at home, everywhere I turn, there is a trace of my wife."

Byung believes that his only alternative to living a "partial life" focused on the loss of Jenny is to realize, "Okay, this is what I have received from God . . . the 'three *T*'s' of time, treasure, and talent," he explained. "I have time, a little bit of talent, and I have a little bit of treasure. I cannot take any of these with me at the end. I will either waste them or I can choose to use them."

In keeping with his convictions, Byung decided to retire soon from his neurology practice of nearly 40 years. The decision has been especially difficult because, he says, "This is my most comfortable place as far as work is concerned. No other place will be like this."

A New Voyage

Byung plans to move to Ethiopia for at least one year and possibly longer after he retires. There he'll continue his previous work at a mission hospital, establishing a clinical neurophysiology service to provide patients with diagnostic testing of brain waves (electroencephalograms) and nerve and muscle function (nerve conduction studies and electromyograms). He's looking forward to "sharing my knowledge, skills, and experiences with somebody who may benefit from them." He reflected that his three "very loving and supportive children want to be grieving and mourning together, but I have decided I should give them a break." He may also consider reapplying to a seminary master's program to which he deferred admission for two years while Jenny was ill.

Byung said that his decision to move to Ethiopia and focus on what he can offer others is something "I have to force myself to do every day. Otherwise I get depressed and downcast."

*"I switched my thinking to look at the bigger picture.
I always desire to live a life that is purposeful to God,
mindful of others, and meaningful to myself."*

Health History

Family medical history: Byung has no family history of memory problems. His mother died at age 66, and his father died at 77.

Medical history: Byung has slightly elevated cholesterol that has been well controlled for many years. He has no major health problems and does not smoke. He follows a "vitality" program through his insurance company that allows him to earn points for maintaining good health and engaging in healthy behaviors.

Brain Health Highlights

Memory function: Byung experiences infrequent word-finding difficulties and no memory problems. He feels he has particularly good recall of details about his patients. His children have told him he has a "photographic memory." He feels that he needs to "use it or lose it" with regard to his memory and is actively engaged in new learning.

Exercise: For the last two years, Byung has walked two to four miles most days of the week. For several years previously, he walked on a treadmill for 30 to 45 minutes three times per week.

Activities and cognitive engagement: Byung works as a neurologist, enjoys reading, and stays in touch with his family by phone, text, e-mail, and visiting.

Diet: Every week, Byung eats six or more servings of dark green leafy vegetables, four or more servings of omega-3 fatty acids (particularly walnuts), and three to four servings of berries. He has at least one serving of whole grains each day and eats no processed foods. He does not drink alcohol.

Sleep: Byung sleeps five to six hours a night and feels well rested about half the time.

Mood: Byung has been very sad since the passing of his wife, Jenny, in November 2018. He keeps moving forward by focusing on "past grace" and looking forward to "future grace." He experiences stress as a result of retiring from his current medical practice, selling his home, and preparing for his upcoming move to Ethiopia.

Social engagement: Byung enjoys spending time with his children, attending church, and participating in short-term mission trips.

Top brain-health habit: Byung starts each day with a devotional and prayer in the morning, which he feels improves his overall outlook.

Advice to others who wish to strengthen their brain health: "Stay active physically, mentally and socially; eat right; and get enough sleep.

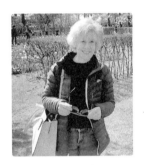

Sue

AGE: 83 (birth date 1936)
BIRTHPLACE: Baltimore County, Maryland
OCCUPATION: Special education teacher

Every weekday around 3 or 4 a.m., before the sun rises, Sue begins her morning routine of reviewing stock market updates, watching premarket coverage, and reading the *Wall Street Journal* "cover to cover" as she prepares to track the market for the day. "There are so many important changes in the market in the early morning, prior to noon," she explained, noting how exciting it is to "delve into the interplay of the companies themselves, what they do, how they affect our economy, and how they compete and integrate with each other." For the last five years, Sue has managed investments for herself and her daughters, and she is hooked on the excitement of it. "My first love is investing," she exclaimed. "My happiest times are when I wake up and I start my day. . . . I love my routine so much."

"My glass is always half full. I'm an optimist."

New Creations

Sue's love of investing blossomed somewhat unexpectedly five years ago after the death of her beloved husband, Verne, who, she recalled, "left me with a hole in my heart." After Verne passed way, "it was like losing my right arm." She remembered feeling like the walls were closing in on her and that she needed to do something about it. There were no readily available community activities for Sue, and she wasn't interested in going the senior living route. "Too institutionalized," she said. "I'd feel my wings were clipped." Instead, she built a new life around all the things she loved. "Not easy at first," she noted, "but what I'm doing now is a distillation of what I set out to do."

When Sue reflected on how she has both persisted and thrived during challenging times, she mentioned that God has been vital to her. "When I was growing up, my mother used to sing a song which still plays through my head," she explained. "'In the Garden.' And yes, 'He walks with me and He talks with me and He tells me I am his own.' Each day. My support system!"

Cherishing Others

Sue is fulfilled by serving others and prioritizes doing that. "The greatest gift is how good I feel when I can do some good each day," she said. Sue reads to three- to five-year-old children several hours a week and enjoys tracking down specific books for them, an extension of the work she loved as a special education teacher. She waited to retire until age 72, noting, "I taught for as long as I could because I loved it so much."

Sue cherishes her time volunteering with older adults. "On Sundays, I go to visit my friends at the nursing home. I bring them chocolates.

I take them mandarin oranges. I bring them books," she said. "There's one man who loves his little bag of potato chips, and we talk. You know, that's my church. It's just reaching out to others, and I have such a good feeling after I return. I have such a good feeling when I'm with them, because I know that they're terribly lonely."

Sue also loves traveling, gardening, cooking, politics, and spending time with her three "amazing" daughters.

Sue describes herself as a determined person, and her tenacity was particularly helpful three years ago when she was diagnosed with Type II diabetes. Instead of taking medication, Sue researched how she could change her lifestyle. She eliminated all sweets from her diet and increased her walking from three miles a day to four miles. Within three months, her blood sugar normalized and she reversed her diabetes. "It took a lot of relentless behavior," she said. "But I did it."

In the summer of 2019, Sue considered taking a few hours off from investment management to get back to playing tennis. For now, though, she laughed, "I do enjoy playing tennis, but I enjoy investing much more."

Health History

Family medical history: Sue has two close relatives with memory problems.
Medical history: Sue was diagnosed with Type II diabetes three years ago but was able to reverse it within three months through exercise and diet. She quit smoking cigarettes 40 years ago.

Brain Health Highlights

Memory function: Sue notices mild problems with word finding and remembering names but says she and her children believe her memory is normal for her age. "I try to keep track of names and try to build my vocabulary constantly," she says.
Exercise: Sue began exercising regularly at age 73, walking three miles per day. She increased her walking to four miles per day three years ago

and uses a fitness tracker to track her distance. She previously played tennis twice a week and would like to get back to it more consistently.

Activities and cognitive engagement: Every day Sue analyzes the stock market for 12 hours, reads the *Wall Street Journal*, and watches world news and business news. She enjoys gardening, watching tennis, reading, and cooking and is "tremendously into politics." She used to paint regularly.

Diet: Each day, Sue eats spinach salad, cruciferous vegetables (broccoli or cauliflower), almonds, strawberries and other fruits, and whole-grain rice and pasta. She has one glass of wine (mostly red) nightly and wild-caught fish one or two times a week. She has not eaten sweets or dessert for the last three years, when she eliminated them to treat diabetes.

Sleep: Sue sleeps five to six hours per night, naps periodically, and generally feels well rested.

Social engagement: Sue enjoys spending time with her family, traveling, and volunteering with children and older adults.

Mood: "I've always been a very happy person."

Top brain health habit: "Exercise. It's not just physical; it's mental and emotional."

Advice to others who wish to strengthen their brain health: "It's important to feel good about yourself physically, mentally, and emotionally. It's important to exercise and eat healthy foods. Reach out to other people. Follow your interests, whatever that might be . . . wherever that might take you."

CHAPTER 10

Meet Your Brain Health Hall of Famers: High-Octane Brain Role Models Ages 91 to 103

"I am still every age that I have been."

—MADELEINE L'ENGLE

This chapter features interviews with four High-Octane Brain "Hall of Famers" from ages 91 to 103. As this book was being written, many people I told about the Hall of Famer interviews were so inspired by them that I interviewed two—rather than one—Hall of Famer in each decade in order to share a wider variety of their stories. Similar to the younger High-Octane Brain role models, the Hall of Famers each reported high levels of brain-healthy habits across most of the five steps in the EXCELS Method.

I often share insights from the Hall of Famers with people in their sixties, seventies, and eighties who say they feel "too old" to achieve more or don't know what else is possible for them as they age. I also love sharing Hall of Famer stories with younger adults who want real-life examples of uplifting men and women who have lived long, adventurous lives, and who have thrived—often, in spite of great challenge. I hope the Hall of Famers also touch your heart and inspire you on your brain health journey!

Otto

AGE: 91 (birth date 1927)
BIRTHPLACE: Cologne, Germany
OCCUPATION: Pastry chef

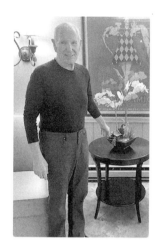

It was a rainy Sunday afternoon in April 2019 when I first met Otto at his apartment in a suburb of Milwaukee, Wisconsin. In our brief telephone call before our interview, he told me in a German accent that his Jewish family survived the Holocaust, that he was a veteran of the navy in World War II, and that he served in the merchant marine. Though I had heard that his youthful appearance and spunky attitude were inspiring to those who knew him, I was not fully prepared to see him striding briskly toward me in the hallway, looking decades younger than his 91 years. ("I could pass for 89," he later joked.)

Otto welcomed me heartily, gave me a tour of his apartment, and proudly showed me several pieces of artwork as jazz played in the background. He also showed me his grandmother's yellow Star of David, which European Jews were required to wear during World War II. He served me cherry pastries as we sat down at a small dining room table to chat.

Otto explained that he and his family were German Jews, that he was an only child, and that his family had worked as bakers. He remembered a time in his childhood when his world changed forever. "This was the ninth of November 1938. It's called the Crystal Night [Kristallnacht, the Night of Broken Glass]," he said. "They got all the Jews. Men at that time. Everybody over 14. They smashed all the Jewish shops . . . that's why they call it the Crystal Night. They broke all the crystal. Every synagogue, which were beautiful, 500 years old, they burned all the synagogues. I went to a Jewish school . . . very, very modern . . . they burned that to the ground." He remembered that fire trucks prevented the flames from the burning synagogue and school from spreading to neighboring buildings.

A Long Way from Home

Otto described his father as "one of the best amateur swimmers in Germany." He was sent to Dachau concentration camp after Kristallnacht. Had it not been for a fortuitous prior event, his father might not have been released. "Two months before, he was walking along [the Rhine River]," Otto recalled. "He sees a boat turn over; the guy apparently was drowning. Jumps in, saves him, brings him on shore. He was one of the top Nazis in the city. So when he was in Dachau, my mother of course went up to him and he helped [my father] get out. We had papers to come to the States for 10 years. He never wanted to go. My uncle and my grandmother and grandfather went to Holland 10 years before. They knew what was coming. The only thing was when the Nazis came into Holland in 1940, all those people who thought they were safe, they all got on the train and went straight to Auschwitz. The gas chamber. Uncle, aunt . . . nice, nice people."

In 1939, Otto and his family "landed in Hoboken, New Jersey, with 20 dollars, not one word of English," and had to start all over again. His father worked at a bakery called Regina's, eventually buying out the owners. In 1944, when Otto was 16, his father died of a heart attack. "I quit school," he said. "I ran the business with my mother."

After working with his mother, Otto served in the navy. "My first love was the Boy Scouts," he recalled. "When I went into the service, I was a little more prepared than anyone else mentally and physically." After serving in World War II and with aid from the GI Bill, he completed culinary school in New York, earning summa cum laude honors, and also attended culinary school in Chicago. He is grateful for the opportunities that America provided him. "I love being an American," he said. "I think I earned my citizenship."

Love in a New City

"I love Milwaukee. I came here 60 years ago for a vacation, and I stayed." It was in Milwaukee that he met and married his beloved wife, Eleanor. Together they ran a premier bakery named Regina's in honor of his father's bakery. They had a son, Michael, of whom Otto is very proud. After Eleanor died in 2001, Otto retired. He said Eleanor was "10 times smarter than I was" but wasn't able to fulfill her dream of becoming a physician because she could attend only three years of school because of the war.

"I don't know why I didn't fall apart after my wife died," Otto said. But a few years after Eleanor's death, he became a caregiver for a woman with Alzheimer's disease, which he found challenging. Since she passed on, he has been hoping to find another companion and is considering joining a dating service. "Sense of humor is my number one," he said, laughing.

"My sense of humor . . . that's kept me going."

Health History

Family medical history: Otto's father died of a heart attack at age 46, and his mother died at age 72.

Medical history: Otto has a history of high blood pressure. He has never smoked.

Brain Health Highlights

Memory function: Otto does not have memory concerns and says that no one has expressed concerns about his memory. "I think I'm 38 years old," he declared.

Exercise: Otto started exercising at age 72, after he retired. Since then, he has been exercising 1.5 hours per day, seven days per week. "My routine is usually I hop on a bicycle for 20 minutes, then I lift some weights and I go on a rowing machine. And then I go on the treadmill and more weights."

Activities and cognitive engagement: Politics, watching television, reading the Sunday paper. "I'm very well versed on finance and the stock market," he said.

Diet: Otto eats a bowl of oatmeal for breakfast and regularly eats whole-grain breads and crackers. He eats fish once a month. He also enjoys a piece of pound cake every day ("I've got a sweet tooth") and one shot of cognac every night (Napoleon French brandy).

Sleep: Otto sleeps eight to nine hours per night and feels well rested.

Social engagement: Otto spends time with friends (including a close friend, Michael, who he feels is like a second son).

Top brain health habit: Exercise. "That is my main thing to keep me going. Physical and mental. I'm the oldest guy at that club [the Wisconsin Athletic Club]," he announced. "They tell me I'm a role model. I never had to force myself to do this. I'm always looking for the next date to go there."

Advice to others who wish to strengthen their brain health: "You have to do it, to get off your keister."

Bill

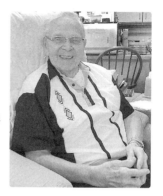

AGE: 93 (birth date 1925)

BIRTHPLACE: Milwaukee County, Wisconsin

OCCUPATION: Building and engineering

A few minutes after I called Bill to schedule an interview, he texted me a confirmation of our appointment. I later learned that he loves technology and spends time every day on Facebook, e-mail, and YouTube on his laptop and smart tablet. He feels that technology helps him accomplish two of his priorities: keeping in touch with his family and friends and staying informed.

Bill was the youngest of six children. He recalled, "We probably were poor, but we didn't know it." He served in World War II, earned a bachelor's degree in building and engineering, and retired at age 62 after working as a construction planner. He technically has four children, but "actually I have five because I kind of adopted a daughter," he explained. "When I was in my sixties I retired, and I went to an aerobics class—I was in aerobics for 10 years—and I met this girl, Laurie, in there. She was my instructor, and we became friends. And to this day she calls me 'Dad' and I call her 'Daughter.' And I have her over for dinner once a month, and I cook for her. She's a very good friend. My best friend. We talk pretty much every day."

Resilience in Action

Three weeks before our interview, Bill had a seventh hip repair operation. He was wearing a hip brace and awaiting another repair of the same hip three weeks after our interview. He continued to walk every day to increase the likelihood of a faster recovery from his upcoming surgery.

On what is important to him, Bill said: "First of all, I have four priorities—God, children, friends, and love of mankind. I wake up in the morning—I do this every morning—I say, 'This is going to be a good day.' The sun is shining. If it's not shining here, it's shining somewhere. It's always shining. Is life hard? Yes. Does life throw you a couple of curve balls? Yes. But you can get around them."

Bill mentioned a major challenge when he was widowed seven years ago after 67 years of marriage. He remembered that after his wife passed, "the first three months, I visited the grave every day. [After] six months . . . Laurie, she called me. She said 'You keep telling me you're going to invite us over for dinner, but you never do. We're coming over Thursday.' That changed my life. I started to live again. Okay, life goes on. You can't just keep moping along. We're all headed to the same path anyway. Some are taken early, some are taken later. You don't know why. But you have to live your life, and the busier you become, the better off you are, so that's when I started volunteering. It's fun to help others because you get to meet so many nice people."

"I'm happy on purpose."

"I Changed My Attitude"

Bill recalled other challenges, including a quadruple bypass, bad knees, and bad hips. "You just live with them," he said. When asked how he was able to thrive in the context of challenges, he explained, "Partly on my own, partly my kids." He said that recently "I had a bad attitude about the care I was getting [at a facility]. And my kids kind of set me straight and said, 'Dad, live with what you got. This is your life. That's the way it's going to be, so change your attitude.' And I thought about that at night, and they were absolutely right. I was feeling sorry for myself, which got me absolutely nowhere, so I changed my attitude."

"God says, 'Love your enemies,'" Bill said, smiling. "Sometimes it's pretty hard to do, but you do it."

Health History

Family medical history: Bill has no family history of memory problems. His father died of a heart attack at age 50, when Bill was 7 years old, and his mother died at age 77. All of his siblings are deceased.

Medical history: Bill has a history of high blood pressure, high cholesterol, quadruple bypass in his fifties, shoulder surgery, ear surgeries to treat hearing problems, and double knee and hip replacements. Bill has never smoked.

Brain Health Highlights

Memory function: Bill does not have memory concerns and says no one has expressed concerns about his memory. His children believe his memory is "incredible," and he shared an example: "When I moved out of my house, I moved my entire workshop into my daughter's house. I built shelves and had everything organized in boxes and in bins. Every time my daughter needs something, I can tell her what wall, what tier, what box, what to look for. If it was in a box mixed with something else, I could tell her that." Bill estimated that he knows the location of items in at least 100 storage bins.

Exercise: Bill started exercising at age 62, after he retired, and attended aerobics classes until age 72. "I loved aerobics," he says, "and especially the step class . . . I was good at it." For the last 21 years, he has walked 5,000 steps per day ("It keeps you active, it keeps you going. It gives you a much brighter outlook on life"). For the last seven years he has been using a recumbent bicycle three times per week for 30 minutes and doing weight training three times a week. He feels that exercise brightens his outlook and "makes me feel I've done something today."

Cognitive engagement: "I love to work with computers." Bill watches the news for 10 hours a day, reads books (in print and digital formats), and spends time on Facebook and YouTube.

Diet: Bill has been eating fish (salmon, tilapia, and catfish) three times per week for the last year and regularly eats nuts (almonds, walnuts), granola with flax seed and oats, and a variety of fruits. He does not eat vegetables ("I hate vegetables") but has one can of vegetable juice a day. He has one alcoholic drink a month when he has dinner with his daughter.

Sleep: Bill sleeps eight hours per night and feels well rested about 90 percent of the time.

Mood: Bill described his mood as "very happy" on most days. He experiences a medium amount of stress and reports high levels of emotional support from others.

Social engagement: Bill volunteers at the store in his apartment community and enjoys spending time with family and friends and watching movies.

Top brain health habit: "Prayer" (for himself and others). Bill tries to follow the "seven-second rule," which he learned recently, and pray for others within seven seconds of learning that they need assistance.

Advice to others who wish to strengthen their brain health: "Exercise first. Second, connect with God."

Caroline ("Carrie")

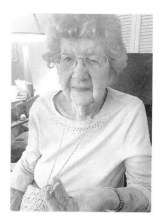

AGE: 100 (birth date 1919)

BIRTHPLACE: Kenosha County, Wisconsin

OCCUPATION: Owned and operated a golf course

Carrie, the third oldest of 13 children, believes that the values she learned on her family's farm were formative to her character and attitude. She recalls cleaning the globes of kerosene lamps, cooking, bottle washing, and taking care of her younger siblings, including a brother who had cognitive delays from meningitis and died at age 22. She remembered that her father's relatives told her mother, "'You should put that boy in a home because that's not good for the other children.' My mother said, 'He is not going anywhere.' And that made us more compassionate in life to help take care of him, which made our lives better."

Carrie dreamed of becoming a nurse but had to leave school in the ninth grade to work at the family farm after the barn burned down, and was never able to return to school. She and her husband had three children and owned and operated a golf course from 1945 to 1959. She recalled that when her husband initially proposed buying the golf course, she told him, "We're young yet, so if we don't make it, we'll start something else." At that time she never expected that she would draw on similar optimism during one of the biggest challenges of her life.

Heartbreak

When her husband was in his late fifties, he began to show symptoms of what later would be diagnosed as Alzheimer's disease. "It finally got to the point where I couldn't keep him in his bed," she recalled. "He started to wander, and that was the part that worried me. He would get out and get on the road or get lost somewhere. He didn't know his children or anything, and it was sad. That was the saddest part of my life." She remembered that when he turned to her one day and asked her, "'Where's Carrie?' I didn't cry about it because I knew it was coming." She was widowed at age 66.

Early on after her husband's diagnosis, "I cried once or twice when I knew what he had. But that didn't help him. It didn't help me," she said. "So I had to start thinking better thoughts. I figure there's going to be a light at the end of the tunnel. Things are going to look better and be better. And they were."

She discussed the importance of moving ahead in spite of hardship. "If something comes up that's really bad, think it out," she said.

"You've got to roll with the punches."

Award-Winning Athleticism

After her husband died, Carrie continued to stay physically active, as she had been since childhood, when her aunt, uncle, and neighbors encouraged her to play baseball. She became an accomplished golfer and bowler, winning 10 golf championships, maintaining a 170-point bowling average for 10 years, and becoming a member of the Racine Women's Bowling Hall of Fame and Golfing Hall of Fame. "So when I got to be 90, I quit bowling and I quit golfing because I felt I did it all," she explained. She continued to exercise, walking regularly, until age 97, when she began to experience balance problems. She has walked with a cane and a walker for the last few years.

For her hundredth birthday in early 2019, Carrie was honored by over 150 people at a 1920s-themed party at a local bar owned by her family. When asked how she has thrived over the years, she leaned over to show me the mother-child figurine on her necklace, pictured above on page 197, which reads, "Don't Worry. Be Happy." Then she laughed, noting that there was one other important thing that she and her daughter do together. "We have a ritual every day, which is another thing that keeps me going. We have a five o'clock cocktail. I have a vodka martini on the rocks."

Health History

Family medical history: Carrie has no family history of dementia. Her father died at age 60, and her mother died at 96.

Medical history: High blood pressure, two small strokes in the last eight years with good recovery, balance problems, and left cornea shrinkage. She has never smoked.

Brain Health Highlights

Memory function: Carrie does not experience any problems with word finding and believes her memory is strong. She says her family members "all brag about how good my memory is" and tell her, "If you want to know something or somebody's name, just ask Carrie."

Exercise: Carrie was physically active from childhood until age 97 and was a championship bowler and golfer (she golfed three to four times per week, bowled twice a week, and walked for many years).

Cognitive engagement: Carrie believes that her brain health is largely determined by her actions and habits. She is very engaged in new learning and very curious. She enjoys watching a variety of television programs (news, *The View, Jeopardy, Wheel of Fortune, Animal Planet,* and various sports, including golf, football, Wisconsin Badger basketball, and the Green Bay Packers). She taught ceramics for 20 years.

Diet: Every week, Carrie has one serving of fish, three to five servings of dark green leafy vegetables, and two to three servings of berries. She eats two servings of whole grains per day and two to three processed foods per week.

Sleep: Carrie sleeps seven or more hours per night and always feels well rested.

Social engagement: She enjoys spending time with her children and other family members. She has lived with her daughter for the last eight years.

Top brain health habit: "Pray. It just gives me a lift for some reason. It just makes me feel better. . . . God is everywhere. I've got plenty of people to pray for, which I think helps. I feel they should have the best that there is too."

Advice to others who wish to strengthen their brain health: "Don't worry. Be happy. You've got to think positive in life. There's ups and downs, and maybe some people have more downs, so it's harder to get back up, but I would say keep a bright side of life . . . be funny once in a while."

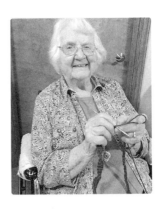

Edna

AGE: 103 (birth date 1915)
BIRTHPLACE: Oconto County, Wisconsin
OCCUPATION: Farmer

Born on a dairy farm, Edna recalled traveling in a horse and buggy for piano lessons at age 12 and boarding away from home to earn a high school degree. Edna was widowed in her sixties after 47 years of marriage and again at age 95 after 24 years in a second marriage. She managed her family's 67-acre farm, filling it with gardens of prized flowers. At age 99, she was given just a few days to live because of an infection after surgery to implant a pacemaker. At that time, her family prepared to share the following poem, which she had written at age 95 for the back of her own funeral card:

Is it really that essential

in one's allotted gift of time

To reach your full potential

For life to be sublime?

I've been a loved and loving wife,

A happy loving mother.

I covet not another life.

I envy not one other.

I count my blessings which are many.

I count my many friends.

I may be down to my last penny

when my earthly lifetime ends.

If I have left some empty space and should someone chance to say

"The world became a better place because she came this way,"

Then that's my measure of success.

I shall not have lived in vain.

If you should ask,

I'd answer "yes" . . .

I would do it all again.

Precious Traditions

Edna laughed as she recalled writing that poem eight years ago. It's one of the hundreds she has written throughout her lifetime, carrying on the tradition started by her great-grandmother, a Civil War bride who wrote poetry for family members as a gift that would "make Christmas last longer" when money was scarce. Edna embraced that tradition, writing poetry to commemorate countless special occasions, including her son's move from home and her second husband's ninetieth birthday.

Family tradition surrounds Edna in the scrapbooks and pictures in her home and is passed down through stories she shares with the many family members who frequently visit her. She also shared the gift of poetry with me, reciting by memory all 36 lines of Rudyard Kipling's poem "If," which she first learned in grade school. She considers "If" a creed for life and has taught it to each of her three children. Her son-in-law proudly explained, "She lives her poetry."

"Take it as it comes"

Joyful Engagement

Edna's talents and interests are vast. She has crocheted and knit afghans, prayer shawls, hats, and baby items for many years; as of early 2019 she had already crocheted 10 prayer shawls since the beginning of the year. She has crafted dozens of commemorative quilts for family members and loves to talk about the stories and symbolism behind their design. She is also highly skilled at cribbage and word games. Her daughter laughed while recalling that higher-skill cribbage players have been sought to play against Edna since she turned age 99 after some in her assisted living community initially underestimated her skills. Her social engagement is a priority to her. She talks to her daughter on the phone every night, e-mails her every morning, and monitors Facebook for family updates.

Edna's zest for life punctuated every aspect of our conversation, and her eyes often twinkled as she spoke about family memories. She frequently joked, explaining, for example, that she likes to tell her daughter that she'll "beam down for a coffee" to her home a few hours away and that the best thing about turning 100 was "a lack of peer pressure."

When asked whether she felt she had overcome any challenges in life, she said she didn't think so. When asked about situations that others might find challenging, such as being diagnosed with colon cancer at age 93, being widowed twice, and almost dying of an infection at 99, she remarked, "It's life."

A few weeks before our visit in May 2019, she wrote and recited a poem for a reading at her assisted living community, noting that the last line was inspired by a similar line from Maya Angelou:

I don't suppose any of us would really recommend
living in a place such as this
while waiting for the end.
But here we are,
in the very same boat,
trying to keep this ship afloat.
So I'll wish you a rainbow
as you sail for the shore.
It's a beautiful day . . .
We've never seen this one before.

Health History

Family medical history: Edna has no family history of memory problems.
Medical history: Edna proudly declared that she was never hospitalized until her eighties. She has a history of high blood pressure, a brain bleed after a fall in her early nineties, diabetes since her early to mid-nineties, colon cancer at age 93 (in remission), knee problems, and a serious infection after the insertion of a pacemaker at 99. Edna has never smoked.

Brain Health Highlights

Memory function: Edna does not have memory concerns or word-finding difficulties. Her daughter and son-in-law report that her memory is excellent and that she easily recalls current information and dozens of poems and events from memory.
Exercise: Edna has used a walker and a wheelchair for a few years because

of knee problems. She propels her walker forward quickly with her feet for a total of 30 to 45 minutes at least four days a week.

Cognitive engagement: E-mail, Facebook, cribbage, word games, writing and reciting poetry, watching the news, discussing politics, and reading (some of her favorites are *Reader's Digest, Our Wisconsin* magazine, and *Chicken Soup for the Soul*).

Diet: Edna has always eaten many fruits and vegetables, a habit she learned while growing up on her family farm. She has watched her diet more carefully since being diagnosed with diabetes in her nineties. She eats fish once a week, dark green leafy vegetables more than six times per week, berries more than four times per week, and whole grains twice daily (including oatmeal every morning). She does not eat processed foods or drink alcohol.

Sleep: Edna sleeps six to seven hours per night and feels well rested.

Social engagement: Edna is in contact with her family every day by phone and e-mail, visits with family and friends several times a week, and monitors Facebook for updates.

Mood: Edna described her mood as "very happy" on most days and her attitude as "easygoing."

Top brain health habit: Generosity. Giving to others makes her happy, which improves other areas of her life. She recalled an impactful situation in which her mother modeled generosity when Edna was a child after some neighborhood girls stole doll dresses that her mother made for her. Her mother went to their home and told them that if they wanted doll dresses, she'd make some for them, and that they didn't have to take them.

Advice to others who wish to strengthen their brain health: "Help everybody you can." She explained how important it is to be generous and support others by spending time with them and doing things for them.

Meredith and Lou: Closing the Circle

Meredith and Lou completed all five steps of the EXCELS Method, and Meredith looked excited as she held up her High-Octane Tracker. Her octane levels for the previous week were in the "Best" range on "**EX**ercise," "**C**onsume," and "**L**ower Stress" and in the "Better" range on "**E**ngage" and "**S**leep."

"The whole really does feel greater than the sum of its parts," she said.

Even though we had discussed the synergy and increased momentum that occur as the habits start to propel one another, Meredith was surprised to experience it personally. This is why it's important to spend only one to two weeks on each of the five steps and move to the next step no matter what your octane level is. Nothing makes the synergy more salient than actually experiencing it, and that synergy often increases motivation to continue the habits. In fact, as Lou had mentioned the previous week, it's common to start feeling that something positive is "missing" if the habits are not continued.

Meredith and Lou were also more consistently using strategies to maximize their octane levels across multiple steps. For example, Meredith prioritized **EX**ercise and **M**indfulness to harness the amplified benefits (see pages 133–36) they provide to mood, sleep, and stress management in addition to their brain-boosting benefits. Lou intentionally chose Multiplier activities that increased his octane levels in multiple categories (such as walking Daisy, which earned him points in "**EX**ercise" and "**E**ngage" and helped improve his "**S**leep" score). You too are encouraged to use Multiplier activities and amplified benefits to experience increased synergy. For an added challenge, see which Multiplier activities you can create to give you the highest number of points across steps. There is no end to the ways you can creatively earn points on the High-Octane Tracker!

Lou's octane levels were in the "Good" range on "**L**ower Stress"; in the "Better" range on "**EX**ercise," "**C**onsume," and "**S**leep"; and in the "Best" range on "**E**ngage." He continued to find it helpful to refer back to the OCTANE acronym ("**O**ne **C**hange at a **T**ime **A**ccomplished **N**ow equals **E**xcellence") at the top of the High-Octane Tracker when he needed to remind himself of the value of the small changes he was making.

"Even two minutes of exercise is better than none," he said when he was asked to paraphrase what OCTANE meant to him. "It took a while for that to sink in, but now it motivates me to just get started . . . and when I do . . . most of the time I keep going. But I really just focus on the start."

The Three-Path Choice works hand in hand with the OCTANE concept: a healthy choice, no matter how small, moves us closer to our Ideal Future Self, our Whys for better brain health, and our High-Octane Brain trajectory. The High-Octane Tracker also helps us tabulate (and celebrate) those healthy choices.

The High-Octane Tracker is designed to be used for the long term as you integrate brain-healthy habits into your lifestyle. Its use is reinforced as you reap the benefits of those habits. Many people use the High-Octane Tracker for a few months until they've firmly integrated brain health into their daily routine. Others (including me) have made the High-Octane Tracker part of daily life and plan to use it for the long term because a system of accountability helps keep brain health top of mind, particularly in the midst of stress and when "life happens." It's also helpful to compare your octane levels on the High-Octane Tracker over time to visualize your progress. Simply keep the original "Steps 1–5" High-Octane Tracker form and scoring pages and make copies as needed.

Completing the High-Octane Tracker with an accountability partner can provide added inspiration and motivation. You might even have differ-ent accountability partners for different steps of the EXCELS Method. For example, you might exercise with one person (or group), do engagement activities with another, and eat brain-healthy foods with yet another.

In addition to enhancing motivation, an accountability partner may help you identify big-picture factors—such as past experiences and personal tendencies—that can unwittingly stall progress. For example, with Lou's help, Meredith recognized that she'd been prioritizing the needs of her clients and family instead of investing time in her future brain health and was then able to shift her behavior and make rapid progress toward her goals.

Meredith in turn encouraged Lou to reengage with the tasks he most enjoyed, like fixing his car, which led him to feel more purposeful in the midst of his grief. Lou's son, Al, even served as an informal accountability partner to Lou. He recognized Lou's disengagement and used their relationship to motivate him to engage in brain-healthy habits. He and Rachel also provided consistent support by making Lou healthy meals throughout the program. If you're not sure whether an accountability partner would be helpful, try working with one and see!

As excited as they were to discuss their progress, Meredith and Lou seemed even more excited to discuss the profiles of the High-Octane Brain role models.

"I've read over these profiles dozens of times," Meredith said, tapping the cover of her binder and shaking her head. "To say I'm inspired would be an understatement. But I was also so touched. . . . These stories are precious, but they also kick me into a higher gear."

"I agree," Lou said. "The role models put the class in a whole new light. It makes it seem more possible to keep this going. Like what we had here wasn't just a fluke that happened because we were helping each other."

"These stories make me see in a new way that brain health creates a healthy life and a healthy life creates brain health," Meredith said. "They feed off one another. It gives me hope . . . maybe I can be a role model someday."

The High-Octane Brain role models expand our understanding of how brain health looks in daily life and provide us with real people to relate to on our journey. They also combat negative societal messages about aging and show us how brain health enriches life regardless of age. Their stories also show us that brain health is uniquely personal and that there is no one way to be successful on the journey. I often think of the role models and am motivated by their resilience and success.

Review the "Top Insights" you noted on your Action Plan while reading the profiles of the High-Octane Brain role models. Who and what stood out to you? Reflect on those highlights to further personalize your High-Octane Brain journey. Personalizing your journey and tailoring it to your life, priorities, and strengths is a major focus of the High-Octane Brain plan. The foundation of this personalization—your unique blueprint—consists of the exercises in your High-Octane Action Plan. Review your answers weekly and update them as your journey evolves so that you stay connected to your motivation. Pay special attention to the Resilience in Action exercise from chapter 7 and remind yourself of your past success under pressure, especially when you need extra motivation.

Meredith, Lou, and I planned to meet again in six months to check in on how they were doing with the program. In the meantime, they planned to stay in touch weekly to share their progress and encouragement.

MEREDITH AND LOU: THE FINAL CHECK-IN

I asked Meredith and Lou to bring an object to their six-month check-in that they felt symbolized their brain health journey. A symbolic object—a picture, a figurine, a plant, or another meaningful item—often has a preexisting positive association and can serve as a salient reminder of progress and boost future motivation.

"Well, that went fast," Lou boomed as he walked into the room. His pace was noticeably quicker.

"Wow, you look great," Meredith said. She'd been on vacation and hadn't seen him for several weeks.

"I'm down about 20 pounds over the last six months," he said, smiling and patting his stomach. As he sat down, he pulled his High-Octane Tracker out of his shirt pocket. "Look at this" he announced, smirking.

The octane levels in all five columns were at the "Better" and "Best" levels, including the "Lower Stress" step, which had always been more challenging for him. He thought his stress was lower because he felt happier and his sleep had improved, which made him feel more relaxed. He'd noticed his sleep got better when he exercised and was notably boosted since he began treatment for sleep apnea. Lou's experience in particular highlights the importance of combining the High-Octane Brain program with personalized medical advice to maximize progress.

Lou also noticed that his memory felt sharper over the previous few months. "It's kind of like I turned back the clock a little," he said. "Al even noticed it. He said I'm remembering our conversations better and more of the information I used to know about cars. He told me he wouldn't have moved if he didn't feel I was getting better. And I feel good about that because I want him to do what's best for him and Rachel."

He explained that Al and Rachel moved out of state after they got married. And though he seriously considered moving with them, he decided not to in the end. "Daisy needs me, and I'd miss my house and my neighbors if I left," he explained. "But it was a tough decision."

Before they moved, Al and Rachel showed Lou how to cook some of the MIND diet recipes they had been making for him. "All I do is make one batch on Sunday and one on Wednesday," he said. "Then I've got my dinners for the whole week. And they do video calls with me every other day. So, you know, they're still keeping an eye on me and giving me pointers . . . and it still kind of feels like they're around."

I noticed that Meredith was beaming as she listened to Lou. "You really motivated me through this whole process, Lou," she said. "Seeing what you could do after all you've been through made me realize I had no excuse not to push my limits."

Meredith was excited that she'd maintained "Better" and "Best" octane levels in all five steps over the last six months. "I'm feeling in the zone. Like I'm getting back to my old self. And I mean my really old self. I'm back at the planetarium for classes every few weeks. I've been gardening and working on my painting," she announced. "I also feel a lot sharper and am less worried about Alzheimer's. I'm doing all I can to fight it, and that feels good. . . . I'm still working hard, but now only part time. And I don't feel guilty about it like I thought I would. I just feel . . . happily busy."

"I know we were supposed to bring an object that was symbolic of our journey," Meredith continued, "but I brought something for Lou. It's just like one I made for myself." Meredith pulled out a small terra-cotta vase and handed it to him. The vase had three white paths painted on it, with a small sunflower at the end of the path on the left.

"I thought this symbolized the journey for me . . . and for us," she said with a smile on her face. "I put some real flowers in it from the new crop in my garden. Speaking of which, my garden is kind of morphing to look like my Ideal Future Self vision, which is good, because it was looking pretty tired before," she said, laughing. "Now I look at it when things get hard, and it reminds me to stick to the journey."

"I did bring one more thing to share, because it reminded me of the changes I've made," she said, pulling a piece of paper from her purse. "This is a poem called 'Love After Love' by Derek Walcott."

She began to read, her voice wavering.

After she finished reading the poem, the room was momentarily silent.

A glint of sunlight shifted slightly behind the blinds. "I've got something you might like, Meredith," Lou said, clearing his throat.

He opened up a picture and beamed as he turned to show it to us.

"It's your Fairlane!" Meredith said excitedly.

"Yup. She's running like a top now. I had to get some help with the repairs, but we're back on the road."

A new High-Octane Brain class would be starting later that day. I asked Meredith and Lou if they had any advice they wanted me to share with the new members.

After a minute Lou leaned forward. "Well, I'd say, 'Look Left. See the High-Octane Brain path whenever you make a decision.' That really helped keep me on track. Oh, and remember," he continued "the tiny changes do add up . . . two minutes is better than zero minutes."

"And I'd say," Meredith added, as she stood up, "at any given moment, we are on a trajectory toward our future brain health . . . and the journey itself changes everything."

Acknowledgments

It has been one of my greatest joys to know, learn from, and be inspired by the incredible people who helped bring this book to life. First and foremost, thank you to the patients I have had the honor to serve. Your questions, needs, and hopes were the inspiration for this book. A million thanks to Linda Konner, my amazing agent: Your wisdom and support have been a beacon on this journey. Heartfelt thanks to Lisa Tener, my book coach, for her invaluable guidance. Hats off to the brilliant editing team at Sterling: Nicole Fisher for championing this book; John Meils, editor extraordinaire and deft shaper of voice; and Barbara Berger, the impeccable conductor who polished countless details to bring this book to life with zeal. Also at Sterling, thanks and admiration to Igor Satanovsky, cover designer, and Gavin Motnyk, interior designer, for the vibrant, engaging design, and to production editor Michael Cea. Thanks also to Robert Johnson for the original Tracker design.

An enormous thanks to the brain health experts for their insights, and the inspiring High-Octane Brain role models; my dynamic colleague Dr. Karen Postal; my cherished "work family" including Paul Mason, Nathalie King, PA-C, Dr. Byung Park, Sally Johnson, Lynette Schroeder, Dr. Janel Schneider, Dr. Bill Bake, Dr. Stephen Pagano, and Matt Barber; my dear colleagues and friends Dr. Amy Friday, Dr. Gina Rehkemper, Dr. Piero Antuono, Tom Hlavacek, Dr. Jessica Chapin, Dr. Brett Parmenter, Dr. Jacqui LoBosco, Dr. Richard Pierce-Ruhland, Dr. Robert Cohen, Dr. Steven Johnson, Dr. John Randolph, the team at the Boston VA and Alzheimer's Association of Wisconsin, Michelle Perri, and Michael Tarney; and my matchless mentors Dr. David Simpson, Dr. David Osmon, Dr. Tom Hammeke, and Dr. Michael McCrea.

Thank you to my beloved family: to my mom for modeling resilience and a Montessori approach to life; my dad for his eternal sunniness; my precious siblings; treasured aunts, uncles, nephews and niece, grandparents, and great-aunt Kathleen; and fetching goldendoodle Rugby. My deepest love and gratitude to my husband Adam: fellow adventurer, household maestro, and doting father to our daughter Halle: the hilarious outer space enthusiast we love beyond measure.

Appendix I

HOW TO USE THE HIGH-OCTANE ACTION PLAN AND TRACKER

The High-Octane Action Plan is your personalized blueprint for better brain health. It provides an at-a-glance review of your answers to the "Reflect" sections in Chapters 1 through 10 (each "Reflect" section includes this thought bubble icon: 💭).

Feel free to update the answers on your Action Plan if they change over time—which is common as the program progresses!

The High-Octane Tracker is your weekly tool for scoring and visually tracking your octane levels as you progress along the five steps of the **EXCELS** Method in part 2 of the book. Tracking details for each step are located in the following chapters, and are highlighted with the word "Track" and this icon: (insert icon)

Step 1 **EX**ercise: Chapter 4

Step 2 **C**onsume Healthy Food: Chapter 5

Step 3 **E**ngage and Learn!: Chapter 6

Step 4 **L**ower Stress: Chapter 7

Step 5 **S**leep for Better Brain Power: Chapter 8

Here are a few tips for using the High-Octane Tracker:

- Most people find it helpful to make a master copy of the High-Octane Tracker before using it the first time, so they can use the forms repeatedly.

- A new High-Octane Tracker is completed each week. However, the first time you go through the program, feel free to do any of the steps for up to two weeks (two tracking forms) before moving onto the next step.

- After Step 1, whatever step of the EXCELS Method you are on should be tracked in conjunction with each previous step. For example, when you track Step 2 (**C**onsume Healthy Food) you will also newly track Step 1 (**EX**ercise) for that same week. When tracking Step 3 (**E**ngage and Learn!), you will also newly track Steps 1 and 2 that same week, and so on with Steps 4 and 5. In other words, your tracking scores for each step will change from week to week (unless you intentionally keep them constant!).

- The gray columns on the High-Octane Tracker (Steps 1 and 3) are scored at the bottom of the tracking page (corresponding octane levels can be shaded in daily). The white columns on the High-Octane Tracker marked with an asterisk (Steps 2, 4, and 5) are scored on pages directly following the Tracker, and the corresponding octane levels are filled in weekly (you will notice that the scoring pages for Steps 2 and 4 are repeated because they are newly scored each week on subsequent steps).

- Your High-Octane Tracker is "complete" for a given week after you've shaded in the octane levels for each step you tracked. This allows you to see all of your octane levels at a glance, and notice how they align with the "Good," "Better," and "Best" categories on the side of the tracking diagram. The octane levels provide you with a visual depiction of your progress incorporating habits that maximize brain health and reduce the risk of Alzheimer's.

Try using your initial octane levels as a "baseline" to compare to future octane levels and to challenge yourself (and your accountability partner if you've chosen to work with one) to gradually increase your octane levels over time. But remember that you are not expected to be perfect across all five steps. The acronym OCTANE (**O**ne **C**hange at a **T**ime **A**ccomplished **N**ow = **E**xcellence) is at the top of your Tracker to remind you of that!

HIGH-OCTANE ACTION PLAN

CHAPTER 2: The Journey Begins

Your "Whys" for Better Brain Health

1. _____

_____

2. _____

_____

CHAPTER 2: The Journey Begins

You "Ideal Future Self"

1. _____

2. _____

3. _____

CHAPTER 3: A Fresh Start

Three-Path Choice

_____

_____

_____

CHAPTER 4: Step 1: *EX*ercise is the X-Factor

Bonus Benefits to Exercise

1. _____

2. _____

3. _____

HIGH-OCTANE ACTION PLAN

CHAPTER 4: Step 1: *EX*ercise is the X-Factor

Joyful Activities

1. _____

2. _____

3. _____

CHAPTER 5: Step 2: **C**onsume Healthy Food

Your Desired Benefit from the MIND diet

1. _____

2. _____

3. _____

CHAPTER 6: Step 3: **E**ngage and Learn!

Appealing Cognitive Activities

1. _____

2. _____

3. _____

CHAPTER 7: Step 4: **L**ower Stress and Boost Well-Being

Positive Stress-Management Tools

1. _____

2. _____

3. _____

HIGH-OCTANE ACTION PLAN

CHAPTER 7: Step 4: *L*ower Stress and Boost Well-Being

Resilience in Action

_____

_____

CHAPTER 8: Step 5: Sleep for Better Brain Power

Top Actions to Improve Sleep

1. _____

2. _____

3. _____

CHAPTERS 9–10: High-Octane Brain Role Models

Top Insights

1. _____

2. _____

3. _____

HIGH-OCTANE TRACKER

One **C**hange at a **T**ime **A**ccomplished **N**ow = **E**xcellence

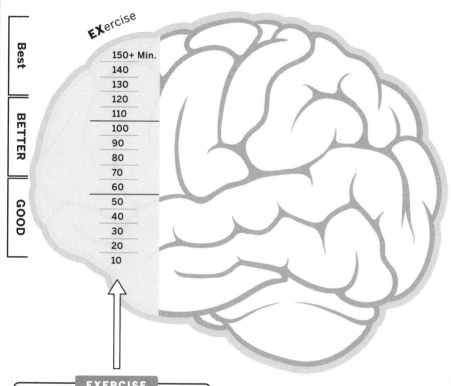

Best

BETTER

GOOD

EXercise

150+ Min.
140
130
120
110
100
90
80
70
60
50
40
30
20
10

EXERCISE

WEEK OF	MIN.	INTENSITY L/M/V
Mon		
Tue		
Wed		
Thu		
Fri		
Sat		
Sun		

Weekly Exercise
Goal (Min)

_____

HIGH-OCTANE TRACKER

One **C**hange at a **T**ime **A**ccomplished **N**ow = **E**xcellence

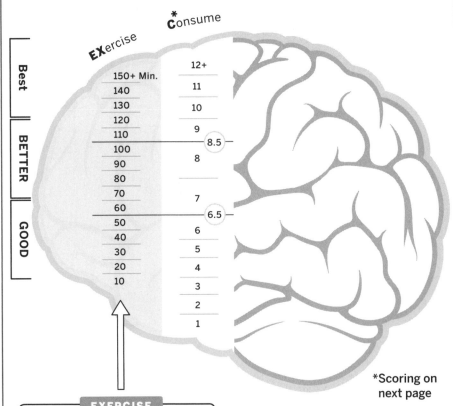

*Consume

EXercise

Best

BETTER

GOOD

	12+
150+ Min.	11
140	10
130	
120	9
110	8.5
100	8
90	
80	
70	7
60	6.5
50	
40	6
30	5
20	4
10	3
	2
	1

*Scoring on
next page

EXERCISE

WEEK OF	MIN.	INTENSITY L/M/V
Mon		
Tue		
Wed		
Thu		
Fri		
Sat		
Sun		

Weekly Exercise
Goal (Min)

_____

CONSUME HEALTHY FOOD

- Over the next week, put a tally mark in the "**DIET COMPONENT**" column for each item that you consume.

- At the end of the week, determine the **MIND** points earned for each Diet Component and write that number in the far right column. Total these **MIND** points at the bottom of the far right column.

- Use this **Weekly MIND Diet Points** total to shade in the OCTANE level on the High-Octane Tracker brain diagram (Consume Column) on the previous page.

MIND DIET COMPONENT SERVINGS AND SCORING

DIET COMPONENT	0 MIND POINTS	0.5 MIND POINTS	1 MIND POINT	WEEKLY POINTS
GREEN LEAFY VEGETABLES	<2 servings/wk	>2 to <6 svgs./wk	>6 svgs./wk	
OTHER VEGETABLES	<5 servings/wk	5 to <7 svgs./wk	>1 svg./day	
BERRIES	<1 serving/wk	1 svg./wk	>2 svgs./wk	
NUTS	<1 serving/mo	1 svg./mo to <5 svg./wk	>5 svgs./wk	
OLIVE OIL	Not primary oil		Primary oil used	
WHOLE GRAINS	<1 serving/day	1–2 svgs./day	>3 svgs./day	
FISH (NOT FRIED)	Rarely	1–3 svgs./mo	>1 meal/wk	
BEANS	<1 meal/wk	1–3 meals/wk	>3 meals/wk	
POULTRY (NOT FRIED)	<1 meal/wk	1 meal/wk	>2 meals/wk	
WINE	>1 glass/day or never	1 glass/mo–6 glasses/wk	1 glass/day	
BUTTER, MARGARINE*	>2 T/day	1–2 T/day	<1 T/day	
CHEESE*	7 + servings/wk	1–6 svgs./wk	<1 svg./wk	
RED MEAT AND MEAT PRODUCTS*	7 + meals/wk	4–6 meals/wk	<4 meals/wk	
FRIED FAST FOODS*	4 + times/wk	1–3 times/wk	<1 time/wk	
PASTRIES AND SWEETS*	7 + servings/wk	5–6 svgs./wk	<5 svg./wk	

* = Foods to minimize
Weekly **MIND** Diet Points ⇨

Reproduced with permission from Dr. Martha Clare Morris

HIGH-OCTANE TRACKER

One **C**hange at a **T**ime **A**ccomplished **N**ow = **E**xcellence

EXercise *C**onsume **E**ngage

Best			
	150+ Min.	12+	
	140	11	11+
	130	10	
	120	9	
	110	8.5	
BETTER	100	8	10
	90		9
	80	7	8
	70		
	60	6.5	
GOOD	50	6	7
	40	5	6
	30	4	5
	20	3	4
	10	2	3
		1	2
			1

*Scoring on next page

EXERCISE

WEEK OF	MIN.	INTENSITY L/M/V
Mon		
Tue		
Wed		
Thu		
Fri		
Sat		
Sun		

ENGAGE

 # ACTIVITIES

Weekly Exercise Goal (Min)

_____

CONSUME HEALTHY FOOD

- Over the next week, put a tally mark in the "**DIET COMPONENT**" column for each item that you consume.

- At the end of the week, determine the **MIND** points earned for each Diet Component and write that number in the far right column. Total these **MIND** points at the bottom of the far right column.

- Use this **Weekly MIND Diet Points** total to shade in the OCTANE level on the High-Octane Tracker brain diagram (Consume Column) on the previous page.

MIND DIET COMPONENT SERVINGS AND SCORING

DIET COMPONENT	0 MIND POINTS	0.5 MIND POINTS	1 MIND POINT	WEEKLY POINTS
GREEN LEAFY VEGETABLES	<2 servings/wk	>2 to <6 svgs./wk	>6 svgs./wk	
OTHER VEGETABLES	<5 servings/wk	5 to <7 svgs./wk	>1 svg./day	
BERRIES	<1 serving/wk	1 svg./wk	>2 svgs./wk	
NUTS	<1 serving/mo	1 svg./mo to <5 svg./wk	>5 svgs./wk	
OLIVE OIL	Not primary oil		Primary oil used	
WHOLE GRAINS	<1 serving/day	1–2 svgs./day	>3 svgs./day	
FISH (NOT FRIED)	Rarely	1–3 svgs./mo	>1 meal/wk	
BEANS	<1 meal/wk	1–3 meals/wk	>3 meals/wk	
POULTRY (NOT FRIED)	<1 meal/wk	1 meal/wk	>2 meals/wk	
WINE	>1 glass/day or never	1 glass/mo–6 glasses/wk	1 glass/day	
BUTTER, MARGARINE*	>2 T/day	1–2 T/day	<1 T/day	
CHEESE*	7 + servings/wk	1–6 svgs./wk	<1 svg./wk	
RED MEAT AND MEAT PRODUCTS*	7 + meals/wk	4–6 meals/wk	<4 meals/wk	
FRIED FAST FOODS*	4 + times/wk	1–3 times/wk	<1 time/wk	
PASTRIES AND SWEETS*	7 + servings/wk	5–6 svgs./wk	<5 svgs./wk	

* = Foods to minimize

Weekly **MIND** Diet Points ⇨

HIGH-OCTANE TRACKER

One Change at a Time Accomplished Now = Excellence

EXercise   *C*onsume   **E**ngage   *L*ower Stress

Best   **BETTER**   **GOOD**

EXercise	Consume	Engage	Lower Stress
150+ Min.	12+		
140	11		0
130	10	11+	1
120			
110	9		2
100	8.5		
90	8	10	3
80		9	
70	7	8	4
60	6.5		5
50	6	7	
40	5	6	6
30			
20	4	5	7
10	3	4	8
	2	3	
	1	2	9
		1	10+

*Scoring on next two pages

EXERCISE

WEEK OF	MIN.	INTENSITY L/M/V
Mon		
Tue		
Wed		
Thu		
Fri		
Sat		
Sun		

ENGAGE

ACTIVITIES

Weekly Exercise Goal (Min)

_____

CONSUME HEALTHY FOOD

- Over the next week, put a tally mark in the "**DIET COMPONENT**" column for each item that you consume.

- At the end of the week, determine the **MIND** points earned for each Diet Component and write that number in the far right column. Total these **MIND** points at the bottom of the far right column.

- Use this **Weekly MIND Diet Points** total to shade in the OCTANE level on the High-Octane Tracker brain diagram (Consume Column) on the previous page.

MIND DIET COMPONENT SERVINGS AND SCORING

DIET COMPONENT	0 MIND POINTS	0.5 MIND POINTS	1 MIND POINT	WEEKLY POINTS
GREEN LEAFY VEGETABLES	<2 servings/wk	>2 to <6 svgs./wk	>6 svgs./wk	
OTHER VEGETABLES	<5 servings/wk	5 to <7 svgs./wk	>1 svg./day	
BERRIES	<1 serving/wk	1 svg./wk	>2 svgs./wk	
NUTS	<1 serving/mo	1 svg./mo to <5 svg./wk	>5 svgs./wk	
OLIVE OIL	Not primary oil		Primary oil used	
WHOLE GRAINS	<1 serving/day	1–2 svgs./day	>3 svgs./day	
FISH (NOT FRIED)	Rarely	1–3 svgs./mo	>1 meal/wk	
BEANS	<1 meal/wk	1–3 meals/wk	>3 meals/wk	
POULTRY (NOT FRIED)	<1 meal/wk	1 meal/wk	>2 meals/wk	
WINE	>1 glass/day or never	1 glass/mo–6 glasses/wk	1 glass/day	
BUTTER, MARGARINE*	>2 T/day	1–2 T/day	<1 T/day	
CHEESE*	7 + servings/wk	1–6 svgs./wk	<1 svg./wk	
RED MEAT AND MEAT PRODUCTS*	7 + meals/wk	4–6 meals/wk	<4 meals/wk	
FRIED FAST FOODS*	4 + times/wk	1–3 times/wk	<1 time/wk	
PASTRIES AND SWEETS*	7 + servings/wk	5–6 svgs./wk	<5 svgs./wk	

* = Foods to minimize

Weekly **MIND** Diet Points ⇨

Reproduced with permission from Dr. Martha Clare Morris

LOWER STRESS AND BOOST WELL-BEING

- On a weekly basis, rate these questions about your experiences.
- Please circle your response and write it in the far right column. Total this column to determine your weekly Stress Points total.
- Use this **Weekly Stress Points** total to shade in the OCTANE level on the High-Octane Tracker brain diagram (Lower Stress Column) on page 224.

	NEVER	ALMOST NEVER	SOMETIMES	OFTEN	
How often have you been upset because of something that happened unexpectedly?	0	1	2	3	
How often have you felt that you were unable to control the important things in your life?	0	1	2	3	
How often have you felt confident about your ability to handle your personal problems?	3	2	1	0	
How often have you felt that things weren't going your way?	0	1	2	3	
How often have you felt that you were on top of things?	3	2	1	0	
How often have you felt difficulties were piling up so high that you could not overcome them?	0	1	2	3	

Weekly **STRESS** Points ⇨

HIGH-OCTANE TRACKER

One **C**hange at a **T**ime **A**ccomplished **N**ow = **E**xcellence

EXercise **C***onsume **E**ngage **L***ower Stress **S***leep

Best | BETTER | GOOD

EXercise	Consume	Engage	Lower Stress	Sleep
150+ Min.	12+			
140	11	11+	0	
130	10		1	
120				
110	9		2	5
100	8.5			
90	8	10	3	
80		9		4
70	7		4	
60	6.5	8		
50		7	5	3
40	6	6	6	
30	5			2
20	4	5	7	
10	3	4	8	1
	2	3	9	
	1	2		
		1	10+	

*Scoring on next three pages

EXERCISE			ENGAGE
WEEK OF	**MIN.**	**INTENSITY** L/M/V	**# ACTIVITIES**
Mon			
Tue			
Wed			
Thu			
Fri			
Sat			
Sun			

Weekly Exercise
Goal (Min)

_____

CONSUME HEALTHY FOOD

- Over the next week, put a tally mark in the "**DIET COMPONENT**" column for each item that you consume.

- At the end of the week, determine the **MIND** points earned for each Diet Component and write that number in the far right column. Total these **MIND** points at the bottom of the far right column.

- Use this **Weekly MIND Diet Points** total to shade in the OCTANE level on the High-Octane Tracker brain diagram (Consume Column) on the previous page.

MIND DIET COMPONENT SERVINGS AND SCORING

DIET COMPONENT	0 MIND POINTS	0.5 MIND POINTS	1 MIND POINT	WEEKLY POINTS
GREEN LEAFY VEGETABLES	<2 servings/wk	>2 to <6 svgs./wk	>6 svgs./wk	
OTHER VEGETABLES	<5 servings/wk	5 to <7 svgs./wk	>1 svg./day	
BERRIES	<1 serving/wk	1 svg./wk	>2 svgs./wk	
NUTS	<1 serving/mo	1 svg./mo to <5 svg./wk	>5 svgs./wk	
OLIVE OIL	Not primary oil		Primary oil used	
WHOLE GRAINS	<1 serving/day	1–2 svgs./day	>3 svgs./day	
FISH (NOT FRIED)	Rarely	1–3 svgs./mo	>1 meal/wk	
BEANS	<1 meal/wk	1–3 meals/wk	>3 meals/wk	
POULTRY (NOT FRIED)	<1 meal/wk	1 meal/wk	>2 meals/wk	
WINE	>1 glass/day or never	1 glass/mo–6 glasses/wk	1 glass/day	
BUTTER, MARGARINE*	>2 T/day	1–2 T/day	<1 T/day	
CHEESE*	7 + servings/wk	1–6 svgs./wk	<1 svg./wk	
RED MEAT AND MEAT PRODUCTS*	7 + meals/wk	4–6 meals/wk	<4 meals/wk	
FRIED FAST FOODS*	4 + times/wk	1–3 times/wk	<1 time/wk	
PASTRIES AND SWEETS*	7 + servings/wk	5–6 svgs./wk	<5 svgs./wk	

* = Foods to minimize   Weekly **MIND** Diet Points ⇨

LOWER STRESS AND BOOST WELL-BEING

- On a weekly basis, rate these questions about your experiences.
- Please circle your response and write it in the far right column. Total this column to determine your weekly Stress Points total.
- Use this **Weekly Stress Points** total to shade in the OCTANE level on the High-Octane Tracker brain diagram (Lower Stress Column) on page 227.

	NEVER	ALMOST NEVER	SOMETIMES	OFTEN	
How often have you been upset because of something that happened unexpectedly?	0	1	2	3	
How often have you felt that you were unable to control the important things in your life?	0	1	2	3	
How often have you felt confident about your ability to handle your personal problems?	3	2	1	0	
How often have you felt that things weren't going your way?	0	1	2	3	
How often have you felt that you were on top of things?	3	2	1	0	
How often have you felt difficulties were piling up so high that you could not overcome them?	0	1	2	3	

Weekly **STRESS** Points ⇨

SLEEP FOR BETTER BRAIN POWER

Every morning, rate your answer to the following question:

HOW WOULD YOU RATE THE QUALITY OF YOUR SLEEP LAST NIGHT?

1 = VERY POOR

2 = POOR

3 = FAIR

4 = GOOD

5 = VERY GOOD

Monday	
Tuesday	
Wednesday	
Thursday	
Friday	
Saturday	
Sunday	

- Add up your total points for the week.
- Divide that number by seven . . .
  This is your **WEEKLY SLEEP QUALITY SCORE** _____
- Use this Weekly Sleep Quality Score to shade in the OCTANE level on the High-Octane Tracker brain diagram (Sleep Column) on page 227.

Appendix II

Dr. Melanie Chandler on Treatment of Mild Cognitive Impairment

Dr. Melanie Chandler is the Director of HABIT at the Mayo Clinic in Florida. HABIT (Healthy Action to Benefit Independence & Thinking) includes memory training, cognitive exercise, yoga, wellness education, and support groups for individuals with MCI and their care partners. She and her colleagues have published research showing that HABIT participants report improved daily functioning, mood, and quality of life, among other positive changes, after completing the program. She is currently conducting a clinical trial on HABIT and hoping to expand the number of locations in which the program is offered.

Since there are no medications to treat mild cognitive impairment (MCI), are there ways to treat MCI with behavioral interventions?

"The most evidence exists for physical exercise. When individuals do cardiovascular exercise—they get in their 150 minutes a week—that has an impact on the risk of dementia later in life. But also, when people already have cognitive impairment and start exercising, they've shown some improvements in concentration and thought speed. After the physical exercise, the next nonmedicine intervention with a lot of research is cognitive intervention or training. A lot of it has been in computerized cognitive games. . . . That tends to have the most impact on working memory and on speed of performance.

"There have been some folks leading research into mnemonic training. They've been trying to get beyond just training on a mnemonic task itself to show real-world generalization. Our work in the area of cognitive intervention has been with compensatory memory calendars [a combined calendar and to-do list called the Memory Support System]. Additionally, there is some evidence that when people do support groups and education about the disease, there's some mood improvement in caregivers and in patients. So those are all important behavioral interventions."

What led you and your team to develop HABIT?

"It's a labor of love that came from a place of wanting to help people. I was a postdoc who had just arrived at the Mayo Clinic, and I had done an internship in brain rehabilitation at the Baylor Scott & White Institute of Rehabilitation in Dallas and had wanted to go to the Mayo Clinic to learn about MCI. Glenn Smith ended up being my mentor for research. And we sat down and had this idea to take the rehabilitation work . . . and marry it with his desire to start doing something for these [MCI] patients. I sat down and worked with the occupational therapist who was doing a version of this [the Memory Support System/calendar] in patients with traumatic brain injury, and we adapted it to MCI . . . into something that was portable yet big enough for older folks to use and simplified down to the things we thought they would most benefit from. It grew from a desire to help these patients. As psychologists we know that we can do more to intervene rather than just give a diagnosis and send folks away and see if they get worse.

"We had to overcome a lot of bias at the time—this was 2004: Why would you do rehabilitation with somebody who has a degenerative condition? So we really just had to prove the idea that . . . they could show benefit from taking notes in a particular way to help them with their memory loss. It was taking something well known in a different population and just bringing it over and adapting it for this population because we knew we could have something to offer. And from the calendar, we just starting building in other things that we also knew theoretically made sense, like doing a support group and an education lecture. People always ask at their diagnostic appointments, 'What should I eat? What exercises should I do for my brain?' So we built that into the educational series."

What makes the Memory Support System different from a daily planner or standard calendar?

"It's a lot more detailed. There are two pages for one day. You have your calendar, where you're putting things at a certain time, but you're also consolidating all the other kinds of lists you might have. So your to-do list is on there as well, and your notes. So those little Post-its or stickies or the notepad by the phone—where you might be jotting down a note on a phone call or something—that's all in this one planner. So everything is in the same place so that folks can have confidence that if they need to write something down, this is where it is. That's what makes it different from the standard wall calendar or pocket calendar that folks have. There's room to write a lot more detail, and we teach people to write a lot more detail than they're used to putting down in a calendar."

> "THIS PROGRAM CAME FROM A PLACE OF WANTING TO HELP PEOPLE."

What are some of the benefits of using the Memory Support System?

"We did a randomized controlled trial where everybody got the calendar. . . . Those who we did the training with had improved self-efficacy and, at first, improved memory-related activities of daily living. As time went on and we got out six months, one year, what we saw was a maintenance of function. So kind of an initial boost and then they're back to their baseline. But why that is still significant and important is that the controls [people who were not using the calendar] were showing a natural decline that you would expect in MCI. So what we were promoting is 'This is not going to cure you and make you better' but the maintenance of function. From the caregiver data . . . six months, a year later . . . what you see is less depression and less burden on the caregivers when their partners are using the calendar."

What types of memory-related daily tasks did people with MCI show improvement in after completing HABIT?

"We can tell you qualitatively all the time that we have folks track their medications, and they have confidence that they've checked them off . . . that they're making it to their appointments more often. We get this feedback from their partners. And just the confidence and the lowering of anxiety . . . of being able to know what they have coming next or know, 'Oh, I already got all of that done.'"

Regarding the different HABIT components, could you speak to the selection of yoga as the physical intervention?

"Yes. I think it was two reasons. . . . We saw that as a time when we could do physical exercise and some mindfulness and relaxation training with folks. It was also a more accessible intervention for us just practically speaking . . . we didn't have access to put everybody on treadmills. Plus, we thought it would be more accessible to people with different physical abilities . . . because it's a chair-based yoga. Whereas we couldn't expect all our patients to be able to go walking, we can get the vast majority of them doing chair yoga in our group setting. At the time we picked it, there was very little research out about doing yoga. There was a small study suggesting it could be beneficial. Then there was a tai chi article that came out a couple of years into it that was even more encouraging about cognitive outcomes. But I think we're seeing more and more, especially with our recent trial showing yoga was the strongest [factor] in terms of maintaining activities of daily living after a year.

"And we're mindful that they're not necessarily getting the cardiovascular exercise that's the recommendation, so as part of the wellness series, we also talk about the importance of the cardiovascular exercise and try to get them the 150 minutes per week. . . . We encourage them to individualize it to what they like to do, whether it's swimming or walking or biking or whatever it is, in addition to the yoga."

What is the impact of the HABIT support groups?
"On the patient end, there's definitely, every time, the comment of 'Wow. I'd never even heard of this diagnosis of MCI, and I was definitely the only person I ever knew of that got this diagnosis. And here I am in a room with eight other people who understand what I'm going through.' And for some . . . that's the biggest part of the whole thing, just not feeling alone, that they have some rare disease. And it's not rare, but it's because they'd never heard of it before that it seems very rare to them, and they don't understand it. So to commiserate with other people that are going through it is huge.

"But they're trying to answer very practical questions for themselves at that phase with the group. 'What's going to happen to me? Who should I tell? Should I tell my adult children that this is going on, or will that only upset them? I'm still working; should I tell my boss about this?' Or 'I'm active on this board; should I tell them that I'm having problems?' Practical stuff like planning for the future. 'I watched my mother. I'm pretty sure that this is Alzheimer's for me because I took care of my mom with Alzheimer's disease. I don't want to do that to my husband. How can I not be a burden to my family?'

"And the partners are doing the same things on their end. Most often they're talking about how guilty they feel because they feel like they're losing their patience. They know it's not a good idea to keep saying, 'I already told you that, don't you remember?' And they're fighting all the time, and they are trying to come to terms with the fact that this problem is real. It's not just their partner being difficult, yet they still are losing their patience. But they talk about, again, practicalities like 'My gosh, I don't want to be driving with him anymore. He terrifies me. What have you done to handle that with your husband or your wife?' And getting not just an emotional working through with us as providers but being able for them to share with each other, emotionally and practically, what they've done too.'"

Do you think there is a synergistic effect with the multiple components in HABIT?

"Oh, absolutely. I think this is also where the calendar plays into the other components, having people write down the different things they learn about in the other components. You're learning about the importance of doing something, about monitoring your depression, going to yoga, and stress management. You go into your calendar training, and you're writing that note: 'Call Dr. Smith about getting back in for the psychiatrist appointment.' So they do feed off one another during the day, and they help. And you are processing your depression in a support group. They love the schedule where they have yoga after another component they may find difficult; they go to yoga and decompress. Perhaps they got stressed by the computer games and then went to group or yoga and could talk about that and work through it. So they're really using all the pieces with each other."

What is self-efficacy, and how do your findings highlight its importance?

"I think self-efficacy . . . is your confidence and your ability to do your day-to-day things despite having this memory problem. And improving self-efficacy, really, you feel it at the end of the program. People feel more confident, they feel better about themselves, they don't feel as embarrassed to go out and still participate in their book club that they were starting to shy away from or whatever other engagement because they have the confidence that they're going to be able to do these things."

You and your team have shown that folks who have milder MCI seem to benefit more from HABIT than those with more severe MCI. What is the ideal time for someone with MCI to start HABIT?

"Right away. We have people who will come in to learn more about the program, and they'll say, 'Well, I don't know if it's bad enough for this yet.' We'll say, 'Now is the time, because the catch is, once things get bad enough or whatever you think is bad enough that you really need it . . . by then your ability to learn these new habits can also be impaired. So don't wait to see how much worse this is going to get or how well you cope. Just get in there and start doing the things right away.'"

Do the participants in the groups ever stay in touch after they've completed HABIT?

"Oh, absolutely. We have ongoing support groups in Florida and Arizona where we continue to see a lot of them regularly, but we learn about their friendships outside too. So that is fantastic to see. I can think of a recent one . . . where the couples really hit it off, and every week they are going out and having dinner and playing some of the games that we introduced them to."

Since the HABIT program is only 10 days long, how can people best maintain the healthy behaviors they learn?

"I think just staying in touch with each other has been helpful. We have a weekly blog and a private discussion group for those who've been in HABIT to keep talking with each other afterwards. I think maintenance of the healthy behaviors we teach is just like any other positive behavior change you may try. Think of the diet you may have tried or the exercise program you started. . . . If you fall off the wagon, you can always get back on, right? Just not giving up on it and returning to it whenever you're able to do so. And with the support of other people around you."

HABIT is available at the Mayo sites in Florida, Arizona, and Minnesota. Are you hoping to spread the program to other sites?
"Oh, absolutely. We've had other sites on past grants that are continuing to use pieces of HABIT. The University of Washington . . . Tallahassee Memorial HealthCare. I was at Emory for a few years after I graduated . . . and last I heard, they're still doing the calendar, support groups, and some education. Definitely the goal is to keep building and have a growing consortium of centers doing this to reach more patients.

"I definitely see HABIT as a delivery system for whatever the most recent evidence-based interventions are for MCI. The more centers we can have implementing this type of delivery system, the more we could try to help answer research questions. . . . That's the dream and the vision."

What would you recommend to people with MCI who can't access HABIT directly and would like to follow a similar program on their own?
"Definitely start taking notes and keeping a calendar. Try to put everything in one place. You can re-create something with a commercially available product that's out there with space to write appointments, to-dos, and notes . . . putting everything in the same place and referring to it multiple times a day to make it a habit. And also, when you make choices about doing other behavioral interventions, like physical exercise . . . how do you translate that into action? You need to have a plan in place. . . . In fact, we use the calendar as a kind of behavioral contracting tool. If you write down, 'I'm going to the gym Saturday at 9 a.m.,' then that's what you've committed to. It gets you from contemplation into action with these other healthy habits people want to do. So it's another reason why I think the calendaring is so helpful for people, because it

also is that behavioral contracting, behavioral activation piece of it, as well as a memory tool."

Has your research influenced the way you live your own life?
"Oh, absolutely. . . . I think there's no way you get in front of a bunch of people and talk about doing these healthy things and not feel a little bit guilty if you don't try to do them yourself. So admittedly, every time HABIT comes around, every couple of months . . . my diet vastly improves by about day three of HABIT. But very practically, we all, the directors, use these things [the Memory Support System] . . . because of the practical, prioritized 'I'm only going to do it today to-do list' being so much effective than that running to-do list. But also credibility that you practice what you preach . . . laying it out in front of patients . . . and they can see that you're doing it, too."

Can you share an example of someone who experienced a particularly meaningful benefit from HABIT?
"I had this patient who, one of the reasons she was brought in to get diagnosed in the first place is that her family had come back for the holidays and she had failed to make the favorite dishes that she always made for her children. And this was a key to them, and it emotionally just devastated her because it's how she showed her love. And so one of the things we did in the calendar training was . . . her son's birthday was coming up and she invited him to come to dinner, and she wanted to make him his favorite rolls. And when she got it done, she wrote a note to me about how he enjoyed them and that she had accomplished it. She was so proud that she cried. There have been lots of times when we've impacted medical compliance, gotten bills paid, or done things people more generally might think 'important.' . . . But that one stands out to me because it also points out that what is an important outcome for one person may be very different for another person. We helped this woman show her love to her family the way she wanted to by doing the program."

Notes

Introduction: Your Future Self

1 Müller, S., Preische, O., Sohrabi, H. R., et al. (2018). "Relationship between physical activity, cognition, and Alzheimer pathology in autosomal dominant Alzheimer's disease." *Alzheimer's & Dementia* 14 (11): 1427–37; Brown B. M., Sohrabi, H. R., Taddei, K., et al. (2017). "Habitual exercise levels are associated with cerebral amyloid load in presymptomatic autosomal dominant alzheimer's disease." *Alzheimer's & Dementia* 13(11): 1197–1206; Beckett, M.W., Ardern, C. I., & Rotondi, M.A. (2015). "A meta-analysis of prospective studies on the role of physical activity and the prevention of Alzheimer's disease in older adults." *BMC Geriatrics* 15(9); Solomon, A., Turunen, H., Ngandu, T., et al. (2018). "Effect of the apolipoprotein E genotype on cognitive change during a multidomain lifestyle intervention: A subgroup analysis of a randomized clinical trial." *JAMA Neurology* 75(4): 462–70; Rosenberg, A., Ngandu, T., Rusanen, M., et al. (2018). "Multidomain lifestyle intervention benefits a large elderly population at risk for cognitive decline and dementia regardless of baseline characteristics: The FINGER trial." *Alzheimer's & Dementia* 14(3): 263–70.

2 Hörder, H., Johansson, L., Guo., X., et al. (2018). "Midlife cardiovascular fitness and dementia: A 44-year longitudinal population study in women." *Neurology* 90(15): e1298–1305.

3 Müller et al., "Relationship," 1427–37; Hörder et al., "Midlife cardiovascular fitness and dementia," e1298–1305.

4 Brown, B. M., Sohrabi, H. R., Taddei, K., et al. (2017). "Habitual exercise levels are associated with cerebral amyloid load in presymptomatic autosomal dominant Alzheimer's disease." *Alzheimer's & Dementia* 13 (11): 1197–1206; Hill, E., Goodwill, A. M., Gorelik, A., & Szoeke, C. (2019). "Diet and biomarkers of Alzheimer's disease: A systematic review and meta-analysis." *Neurobiology of Aging* 76: 45–52.

5 Alzheimer's Disease International. *World Alzheimer's Report 2018.* "The state of the art of dementia research: New frontiers." https://www.alz.co.uk/research/WorldAlzheimerReport2018.pdf. Retrieved 8/3/2019.

6 Alzheimer's Association. *2019 Alzheimer's Facts and Figures.* https://www.alz.org/media/Documents/alzheimers-facts-and-figures-2019-r.pdf. Retrieved 8/3/2019.

7 Younes, L., Albert, M., Moghekar, A., Soldan, A., Pettigrew, C., & Miller, M. I. "Identifying changepoints in biomarkers during the preclinical phase of Alzheimer's disease." (2019). *Frontiers in Aging Neuroscience* 11: 74.

8 Cannon-Albright, L. A., Foster, N. L., Schliep, K., et al. (2019). "Relative risk for Alzheimer disease based on complete family history." *Neurology* 92(15): e1745–53.

9 Morris, M. C. *Diet for the MIND.* New York: Little, Brown, 2017.

10 Salthouse, T. A. "When does age-related cognitive decline begin?" (2009). *Neurobiology of Aging* 30(4): 507–14.

11 Raz, N., Lindenberger, U., Rodrigue, K. M., et al. (2005). "Regional brain changes in aging healthy adults: General trends, individual differences and modifiers." *Cerebral Cortex* 15: 1676–89; Jack, C. R., Shiung, M. M., Weigand, S. D., et al. (2005), "Brain atrophy rates predict subsequent clinical conversion in normal elderly and amnestic MCI." *Neurology* 65(8): 1227–31.

12 American Association of Retired Persons (AARP). *2015 Survey on Brain Health.* https://www.aarp.org/research/topics/health/info-2015/2015-brain-health-survey.html. Retrieved 8/3/2019.

Chapter 1 • The High-Octane Brain Revolution

13 Hellmuth, J., Rabinovici, G. D., & Miller, B. L. (2019). "The rise of pseudomedicine for dementia and brain health." *JAMA* 321(6): 543–44.

14 Marist Poll, November 2012 (conducted on behalf of Home Instead Senior Care). http://maristpoll.marist.edu/1114-alzheimers-most-feared-disease/#sthash.o1rmta80.dpbs. Retrieved 12/17/2019.

15 Alzheimer's Disease International. *World Alzheimer's Report 2018.*

16 Brookmeyer, R., Johnson, E., Ziegler-Graham, K., & Arrighi, H. M. (2007). "Forecasting the global burden of Alzheimer's disease." *Alzheimer's & Dementia* 3(3): 186–91.

17 Barnes, D. E., & Yaffe, K. (2011). "The projected impact of risk factor reduction on Alzheimer's disease prevalence." *Lancet Neurology* 10(9): 819–28.

18 Alzheimer's Association and the Centers for Disease Control and Prevention. *Healthy Brain Initiative, State and Local Public Health Partnerships to Address Dementia: The 2018–2023 Road Map*, 2018. https://www.cdc.gov/aging/pdf/2018-2023-Road-Map-508.pdf. Retrieved 8/3/2019.

19 World Health Organization. *Risk Reduction of Cognitive Decline and Dementia: WHO Guidelines*, 2019. https://apps.who.int/iris/bitstream/handle/10665/312180/9789241550543-eng.pdf?ua=1. Retrieved 8/3/2019.

20 Baumgart, M., Snyder, H. M., Carrillo, M. C., et al. (2015). "Summary of the evidence on modifiable risk factors for cognitive decline and dementia: A population-based perspective." *Alzheimer's & Dementia* 11(6): 718–26.

21 Institute of Medicine of the National Academies. *Cognitive Aging: Progress in Understanding and Opportunities for Action*, 2015. https://www.nap.edu/read/21693/chapter/1. Retrieved 8/3/2019.

22 World Health Organization. *Ageing and Health*, 2018. https://www.who.int/news-room/fact-sheets/detail/ageing-and-health. Retrieved 8/3/2019.

23 Bekris, L. M., Yu, C., Bird, T. D., & Tsuang, D. W. (2010). "Genetics of Alzheimer disease." *Geriatriac Psychiatry and Neurology* 23(4): 213–27.

24 Bird, T. D. "Early-onset familial Alzheimer disease." In: Adam M. P., Ardinger, H. H., Pagon, R. A., et al., eds. *GeneReviews.* Seattle: University of Washington, 1993–2019. Available from https://www.ncbi.nlm.nih.gov/books/NBK1236/. Retrieved 8/3/2019.

25 Salthouse, "When does age-related cognitive decline begin?," 507–14.

26 Verhaeghen, P. (2003). "Aging and vocabulary scores: A meta-analysis." *Psychology and Aging* 8(2): 332–39.

27 Fleischman, D. A., Leurgans, S., Arfanakis, K., et al. (2014). "Gray-matter macrostructure in cognitively healthy older persons: Associations with age and cognition." *Brain Structure and Function* 219(6): 2029–49.

28 Fleischman et al., "Gray-matter macrostructure," 2029–49.

29 Querfurth, H. W., & LaFerla, F. M. (2010). "Alzheimer's disease." *New England Journal of Medicine* 362(4): 329–44.

30 Alzheimer's Association. *2019 Alzheimer's Facts and Figures.*

31 Hebert, L. E., Weuve, J., Scherr, P.A., & Evans, D. A. (2013). "Alzheimer disease in the United States (2010–2050) estimated using the 2010 Census." *Neurology* 80(19): 1778–83.

32 Younes et al., "Identifying changepoints," 74.

33 Schneider, J. A., Arvanitakis, Z., Bang, W., & Bennett, D. A. (2007). "Mixed brain pathologies account for most dementia cases in community-dwelling older persons." *Neurology* 69(24): 2197–204.

34 Alzheimer's Association. *2019 Alzheimer's Facts and Figures*; Nelson, P. T., Dickson, D. W., Trojanowski, J. Q., et al. (2019). "Limbic-predominant age-related TDP-43 encephalopathy (LATE): Consensus working group report." *Brain* 142(6): 1503–27.

35 Morris, J. K., Vidoni, E. D., Johnson, D. K., et al. (2017). "Aerobic exercise for Alzheimer's disease: A randomized controlled pilot trial." *PLOS One* 12(2): e0170547.

36 Groot, C., Hooghiemstra, A. M., & Raijmakers, P. G. (2016). "The effect of physical activity on cognitive function in patients with dementia: A meta-analysis of randomized control trials." *Ageing Research Reviews* 25: 13–23.

37 Ginis, K. A., Heisz, J., & Spence, J. C. (2017). "Formulation of evidence-based messages to promote the use of physical activity to prevent and manage Alzheimer's disease." *BMC Public Health* 17(1): 209.

38 Capotosto, E., Belacchi, C., Gardini, S., et al. (2017). "Cognitive stimulation therapy in the Italian context: Its efficacy in cognitive and non-cognitive measures in older adults with dementia." *International Journal of Geriatric Psychiatry* 32(3): 331–40.

39 Gómez, G. M., & Gómez, G. J. (2017). "Music therapy and Alzheimer's disease: Cognitive, psychological, and behavioural effects." *Neurologia* 32(5): 300–308.

40 Kaufman, Y., Anaki, D., Binns, M., & Freedman, M. (2007). "Cognitive decline in Alzheimer disease: Impact of spirituality, religiosity, and QOL." *Neurology* 68(18): 1509–14.

41 Agli, O., Bailly, N., & Ferrand, C. (2015). "Spirituality and religion in older adults with dementia: A systematic review." *International Psychogeriatrics* 27(5): 715–25.

42 National Institutes of Health, US National Library of Medicine. *Multimodal Preventive Trial for Alzheimer's Disease (MIND-ADmini).* https://clinicaltrials.gov/ct2/show/NCT03249688. Retrieved 8/3/2019.

43 Sachdev, P. S., Lipnicki, D. M., Kochan, N. A., et al. (2015). "The prevalence of mild cognitive impairment in diverse geographical and ethnocultural regions: The COSMIC collaboration." *PLOS One* 10(11): e0142388.

44 Baker, L. D., Skinner, J. S., & Craft, S. (2015). "Aerobic exercise reduces phosphorylated tau protein in cerebrospinal fluid in older adults with mild cognitive impairment." *Alzheimer's & Dementia* 11(7): s324.

45 Baker et al., "Aerobic exercise," s324.

46 National Institute on Aging, Alzheimer's Disease Cooperative Study. *Exercise in Adults with Mild Memory Problems (EXERT).* https://www.nia.nih.gov/alzheimers/clinical-trials/exercise-adults-mild-memory-problems-exert. Retrieved 8/3/2019.

47 Singh, B., Parsaik, A. K., Mielke, M. M., et al. (2014). "Association of Mediterranean

diet with mild cognitive impairment and Alzheimer's disease: A systematic review and meta-analysis." *Journal of Alzheimer's Disease* 39(2): 271–82.

48 Farhang, M., Miranda-Castillo, C., Rubio, M., & Furtado, G. (2019). "Impact of mind-body interventions in older adults with mild cognitive impairment: A systematic review." *International Psychogeriatrics* 4: 1–24.

49 Burzynska, A. Z., Wong, C. N., Chaddock-Heyman, L., et al. (2016). "White matter integrity, hippocampal volume, and cognitive performance of a world-famous nonagenarian track-and-field athlete." *Neurocase* 22(2): 135–44.

50 Snowdon, D. A., Greiner, L. H., & Markesbery, W. R. (2000). "Linguistic ability in early life and the neuropathology of Alzheimer's disease and cerebrovascular disease: Findings from the Nun Study." *Annals of the New York Academy of Sciences* 903: 34–8.

51 Snowdon, D. A. (2003). "Healthy aging and dementia: Findings from the Nun Study." *Annals of Internal Medicine* 139(5 Part 2): 450–54.

52 Snowdon, "Healthy aging," 450–54.

53 Snowdon. (1997). "Aging and Alzheimer's disease: Lessons from the Nun Study." *Gerontologist* 37(2): 150–56.

54 Negash, S., Wilson, R. S., Leurgans, S. E., et al. (2013). "Resilient brain aging: Characterization of discordance between Alzheimer's disease pathology and cognition." *Current Alzheimer Research* 10(8): 844–51.

55 Cook, A. H., Sridhar, J., Ohm, D., et al. (2017). "Rates of cortical atrophy in adults 80 years and older with superior vs average episodic memory." *JAMA* 317(13): 1373–75.

56 Gorelick, P. B., Furie, K. L., Iadecola, C., Smith, E. E., et al. (2017). "Defining optimal brain health in adults: A presidential advisory from the American Heart Associa-tion/American Stroke Association." *Stroke* 48(10): e284–303.

Chapter 2 • The Journey Begins

57 Rosenberg et al., "Multidomain lifestyle intervention," 263–70.

58 Kulmala, J., Ngandu, T., Havulinna, S., et al. (2019). "The effect of multidomain lifestyle intervention on daily functioning in older people." *Journal of the American Geriatrics Society* 67(6): 1138–44.

59 Solomon et al., "Effect of the apolipoprotein E genotype on cognitive change," 462–70.

60 Sindi, S., Ngandu, T., Hovatta, I., et al. (2017). "Baseline telomere length and effects of a multidomain lifestyle intervention on cognition: The FINGER randomized controlled trial." *Jounal of Alzheimer's Disease* 59(4): 1459–70.

61 Hörder et al., "Midlife cardiovascular fitness and dementia," e1298–1305.

62 Müller et al., "Relationship between physical activity, cognition, and Alzheimer pathology," 1427–37.

63 Müller et al., "Relationship between physical activity, cognition, and Alzheimer pathology," 1427–37; Brown, B. M., Sohrabi, H. R., Taddei, K., et al. (2017). "Habitual exercise levels are associated with cerebral amyloid load in presymptomatic autosomal dominant Alzheimer's disease." *Alzheimer's & Dementia* 13(11): 1197–1206.

64 Boyle, P. A., Buchman, A. S., Barnes, L. L., & Bennett, D. A. (2010). "Effect of a purpose in life on risk of incident Alzheimer disease and mild cognitive impairment in community-dwelling older persons." *Archives of General Psychiatry* 67(3): 304–10.

Chapter 3 • A Fresh Start: How to Maximize Your Brain Health

65 Wu, L., & Zhao, L. (2016). "ApoE2 and Alzheimer's disease: time to take a closer look." *Neural Regeneration Research* 11(3): 412–13.

66 Bird, "Early-onset familial Alzheimer disease," 1993–2019.

67 Cannon-Albright et al., "Relative risk for Alzheimer disease," e1745-e1753.

68 Cannon-Albright et al., "Relative risk for Alzheimer disease," e1745-e1753.

69 Perani, D., Farsad, M., Ballarini, T., et al. (2017). "The impact of bilingualism on brain reserve and metabolic connectivity in Alzheimer's dementia." *Proceedings of the National Academy of Sciences of the United States of America (PNAS)* 114(7): 1690–95; Woumans, E., Santens, P., Sieben, A., Versijpt, J., Stevens, M., & Duyck, W. (2015). "Bilingualism delays clinical manifestation of Alzheimer's disease." *Bilingualism: Language and Cognition* 18(3): 568–74.

70 Pike, C. J. (2017). "Sex and the development of Alzheimer's disease." *Journal of Neuroscience Research* 95(1–2): 671–80.

71 Alzheimer's Association. *2019 Alzheimer's Facts and Figures.*

72 Alzheimer's Disease International. *World Alzheimer's Report 2015: The Global Impact of Dementia.* https://www.alz.co.uk/research/worldalzheimerreport2015summary.pdf. Retrieved 8/03/2019.

73 Debette, S., Seshadri, S., Beiser, A., et al. (2011). "Midlife vascular risk factor exposure accelerates structural brain aging and cognitive decline." *Neurology* 77(5): 461–68.

74 Weiner, M. W., Crane, P. K., Montine, T. M., Bennett, D. A., & Veitch, D. P. (2017). "Traumatic brain injury may not increase the risk of Alzheimer disease." *Neurology* 89(18): 1923–25; Dams-O'Connor, K., Guetta, G., Hahn-Ketter, A. E., & Fedor, A. (2016). "Traumatic brain injury as a risk factor for Alzheimer's disease: Current knowledge and future directions." *Neurodegenerative Disease Management* 6(5): 417–29.

75 Erickson, K. I, Creswell, J. D., Verstynen, T. D., & Gianaros, P. J. (2014). "Health neuroscience: Defining a new field." *Current Directions in Psychological Science* 23(6): 446–53.

76 Leckie, R. L., Manuck, S. B., Bhattacharjee, N., et al. (2014). "Omega-3 fatty acids moderate effects of physical activity on cognitive function." *Neuropsychologia* 59: 103–11.

77 Recchia, D., Baghdadli, A., Lassale, C., et al. (2019). "Associations between long-term adherence to healthy diet and recurrent depressive symptoms in Whitehall II Study." *European Journal of Nutrition.* doi: 10.1007/s00394-019-01964-z.

78 World Health Organization. *Risk Reduction of Cognitive Decline and Dementia.*

79 Spira, A. P., & Gottesman, R. F. (2017). "Sleep disturbance: An emerging opportunity for Alzheimer's disease prevention?" *International Psychogeriatrics* 29(4): 529–31.

Chapter 4 • EXercise Is the X-Factor

80 Hörder et al., "Midlife cardiovascular fitness and dementia," e1298–1305.

81 Blondell, S. J., Hammersley-Mather, R., & Veerman, J. L. (2014). "Does physical activity prevent cognitive decline and dementia? A systematic review and meta-analysis of longitudinal studies." *BMC Public Health* 14: 510; Hamer, M., & Chida, Y. (2009). "Physical activity and risk of neurodegenerative disease: A systematic review of prospective evidence." *Psychological Medicine* 39(1): 3–11.

82 Defina, L. F., Willis, B. L., Radford, N. B., et al. (2013). "The association between midlife cardiorespiratory fitness levels and later-life dementia: A cohort study." *Annals of Internal Medicine* 158(3): 162–68.

83 Larson, E. B., Wang, L., Bowen, J. D., McCormick, W. C., Teri, L., Crane, P., & Kukull, W. (2006). "Exercise is associated with reduced risk for incident dementia among persons 65 years of age and older." *Annals of Internal Medicine* 144(2): 73–81.

84 Guure, C. B., Ibrahim, N. A., Adam, M. B., & Said, S. M. (2017). "Impact of physical activity on cognitive decline, dementia, and its subtypes: Meta-analysis of prospective studies." *BioMed Research International* 2017: 1–13.

85 Abbott, R. D., White, L. R., Ross, W., Masak, K., Curb, D., & Petrovitch, H. (2004). "Walking and dementia in physically capable elderly men." *JAMA* 292(12): 1447–53.

86 Erickson, K. I., Voss, M. W., Prakash, R. S., et al. (2011). "Exercise training increases size of hippocampus and improves memory." *PNAS* 108(7): 3017–22; Oberlin, L. E., Verstynen, T. D., Burzynska, A.Z., et al. (2016). "White matter microstructure mediates the relationship between cardiorespiratory fitness and spatial working memory in older adults." *NeuroImage* 131: 91–101; Leckie, R. L., Oberlin, L. E., Voss, M. W., et al. (2014). "BDNF mediates improvements in executive function following a 1-year exercise intervention." *Frontiers in Human Neuroscience* 8: 985; Prakash, R. S., Voss, M. W., Erickson, K. I., & Kramer, A. F. (2015). "Physical activity and cognitive vitality." *Annual Review of Psychology* 66: 769–97; Tian, Q., Erickson, K. I., & Simonsick, E. M. (2014). "Physical activity predicts microstructural integrity in memory-related networks in very old adults." *Journals of Gerontology. Series A, Biological Sciences and Medical Sciences (JGABS&MS)* 69(10): 1284–90.

87 Nishiguchi, S., Yamada, M., Tanigawa, T., et al. (2015). "A 12-week physical and cognitive exercise program can improve cognitive function and neural efficiency in community-dwelling older adults: A randomized controlled trial." *Journal of the American Geriatrics Society* 63(7): 1355–63.

88 Colcombe, S. J., Erickson, K. I., Scalf, P. E., et al. (2006). "Aerobic exercise training increases brain volume in aging humans." *JGABS&MS* 61(11): 1166–70.

89 Erickson, K. I., Raji, C. A., Lopez, J. T., et al. (2010). "Physical activity predicts gray matter volume in late adulthood." *Neurology* 75(16): 1415–22.

90 Stillman, C. M., Lopez, O. L., Becker, J. T., et al. (2017). "Physical activity predicts reduced plasma β amyloid in the Cardiovascular Health Study." *Annals of Clinical and Translational Neurology* 4(5): 284–91.

91 Erickson et al., "Exercise training increases size of hippocampus," 3017–22.

92 Stern, Y., MacKay-Brandt, A., Lee, S., et al. (2019). "Effect of aerobic exercise on cognition in younger adults: A randomized clinical trial." *Neurology* 92(9): e905–16.

93 Oberlin, L. E., Verstynen, T.D., Burzynska, A. Z., et al. (2016). "White matter microstructure mediates the relationship between cardiorespiratory fitness and spatial working memory in older adults." *NeuroImage* 131: 91–101; Leckie, R. L., Oberlin, L. E., Voss, M. W., et al. (2014). "BDNF mediates improvements in executive function following a 1-year exercise intervention." *Frontiers in Human Neuroscience* 8: 985; Tian, Q., Erickson, K. I., & Simonsick, E. M. (2014). "Physical activity predicts microstructural integrity in memory-related networks in very old adults." *JGABS&MS* 69(10): 1284–90.

94 Spartano, N. L., Davis-Plourde, K. L., Himali, J. J., et al. (2019). "Association of accelerometer-measured light-intensity physical activity with brain volume: The

Framingham Heart Study." *JAMA Network Open* 2(4): e192745; Cabral, D. F., Rice, J., Morris, T. P., Rundek, T., Pascual-Leone, A., & Gomes-Osman, J. (2019). "Exercise for brain health: An investigation into the underlying mechanisms guided by dose." *Neurotherapeutics* 16(3): 580–99.

95　Shaaban, C. E., Aizenstein, H. J., Jorgensen, D. R., et al. "Physical activity and cerebral small vein integrity in older adults." *Medicine & Science in Sports & Exercise* 51(8): 1684–91.

96　Cabral et al., "Exercise for brain health," 580–99.

97　Leckie et al., "BDNF mediates improvements in executive function," 985; Colcombe, S., & Kramer, A. F. (2003). "Fitness effects on the cognitive function of older adults: A meta-analytic study." *Psychological Science* 14(2): 125–30.

98　Leckie et al., "BDNF mediates improvements in executive function," 985.

99　Cabral et al., "Exercise for brain health," 580–99.

100　Rebelo-Marques, A., De Sousa Lages, A., Ribeiro, C. F., Mota-Pinto, A., Carrilho, F., & Espregueira-Mende, F. (2018). "Aging hallmarks: The benefits of physical exercise." *Frontiers in Endocrinology (Lausanne)* 9: 258.

101　Cabral et al., "Exercise for brain health," 580–99.

102　Colcombe & Kramer, "Fitness effects on the cognitive function of older adults," 125–30.

103　Stillman et al., "Physical activity predicts reduced plasma β amyloid," 284–91.

104　Tucker, J. M., Welk, G. J., & Beyler, N. K. (2011). "Physical activity in U.S.: Adults compliance with the Physical Activity Guidelines for Americans." *American Journal of Preventive Medicine* 40(4): 454–61.

105　Spartano et al., "Association of accelerometer-measured light-intensity," e192745.

106　Spartano et al., "Association of accelerometer-measured light-intensity," e192745.

107　Buchman, A. S., Boyle, P. A., Yu, L., Shah, R. C., Wilson, R. S., & Bennett, D. A. (2012). "Total daily physical activity and the risk of AD and cognitive decline in older adults." *Neurology* 78(17): 1323–29; Bangsbo, J., Blackwell, J., Boraxbekk, C. J., et al. (2019). "Copenhagen consensus statement 2019: Physical activity and ageing." *British Journal of Sports Medicine* 53(14): 856–58.

108　Bangsbo et al., "Copenhagen consensus statement 2019," 856–58.

109　Bangsbo et al., "Copenhagen consensus statement 2019," 856–58; McSween, M. P., Coombes, J. S., MacKay, C. P., et al. (2019). "The immediate effects of acute aerobic exercise on cognition in healthy older adults: A systematic review." *Sports Medicine* 49(1): 67–82.

110　Piercy, K. L., Troiano, R. P., Ballard, R. M., et al. (2018). "The Physical Activity Guidelines for Americans." *JAMA* 320(19): 2020–28.

111　Piercy et al. "The Physical Activity Guidelines for Americans," 2020–28.

112　Roig, M., Thomas, R., Mange, C. S., et al. (2016). "Time-dependent effects of cardiovascular exercise on memory." *Exercise and Sport Sciences Reviews* 44: 81–88.

113　World Health Organization. *Risk Reduction of Cognitive Decline and Dementia*; Piercy et al. "The physical activity guidelines for Americans," 2020–28; Powell, K. E., King, A. C., Buchner, D. M., et al. (2018). "The Scientific Foundation for the Physical Activity Guidelines for Americans," 2nd ed. *Journal of Physical Activity and Health* 17: 1–11.

114　World Health Organization. *Risk Reduction of Cognitive Decline and Dementia*; Piercy et al. "The Physical Activity Guidelines for Americans," 2020–28.

115　Piercy et al. "The Physical Activity Guidelines for Americans," 2020–28.

116　Powell et al. "*The Scientific Foundation for the Physical Activity Guidelines,*" 1–11.

Chapter 5 • Consume Healthy Foods

117 AARP, *2015 Survey on Brain Health.*

118 Estruch, R., Ros, E., & Salas-Salvado, J. (2013). "Primary prevention of cardiovascular disease with a Mediterranean diet." *New England Journal of Medicine* 368(14): 1279–90.

119 Morris, M. C. (2004). "Diet and Alzheimer's disease: What the evidence shows." *Medscape General Medicine* 6(1): 48.

120 Valls-Pedret, C., Sala-Vila, A., Serra-Mir, M., et al. (2015). "Mediterranean diet and age-related cognitive decline. A randomized clinical trial." *JAMA Internal Medicine* 175(7): 1094–03.

121 Hill et al., "Diet and biomarkers of Alzheimer's disease," 45–52; Chen, X., Maguire, B., Brodaty, H., & O'Leary, F. (2019). "Dietary patterns and cognitive health in older adults: A systematic review." *Journal of Alzheimer's Disease* 67(2): 583–619; Klímová, B., & Vališ, M. (2018). "Nutritional interventions as beneficial strategies to delay cognitive decline in healthy older individuals." *Nutrients* 10(7). pii: E905; Solfrizzi, V., Custodero, C., Lozupone, M., et al. (2017). "Relationships of dietary patterns, foods, and micro- and macronutrients with Alzheimer's disease and late-life cognitive disorders: A systematic review." *Journal of Alzheimer's Disease* 59(3): 815–49.

122 Solfrizzi et al., "Relationships of dietary patterns," 815–49.

123 Morris, *Diet for the MIND.*

124 Van den Brink, A. C., Brouwer-Brolsma, E. M., Berendsen, A. A. M., & van de Rest, O. (2019). "The Mediterranean, Dietary Approaches to Stop Hypertension (DASH), and Mediterranean-DASH Intervention for Neurodegenerative Delay (MIND) diets are associated with less cognitive decline and a lower risk of Alzheimer's disease: A review." *Advances in Nutrition* June 18. pii: nmz054. doi: 10.1093/advances/nmz054. [Epub ahead of print]

125 Valls-Pedret et al., "Mediterranean diet and age-related cognitive decline," 1094–03; Smith, P. J., Blumenthal, J. A., Babyak, M. A., et al. (2010). "Effects of the dietary approaches to stop hypertension diet, exercise, and caloric restriction on neurocognition in overweight adults with high blood pressure." *Hypertension* 55(6): 1331–38.

126 Morris, *Diet for the MIND.*

127 Morris, *Diet for the MIND.*

128 Morris, *Diet for the MIND.*

129 AARP Global Council on Brain Health (2019). *The Real Deal on Brain Health Supplements: GCBH Recommendations on Vitamins, Minerals, and Other Dietary Supplements.* Available at www.GlobalCouncilOnBrainHealth.org. https://doi.org/10.26419/pia.00094.001.

130 AARP. *2019 AARP Brain Health and Dietary Supplements Survey.* https://www.aarp.org/content/dam/aarp/research/surveys_statistics/health/2019/brain-health-and-dietary-supplements-report.doi.10.26419-2Fres.00318.001.pdf. Retrieved 8/3/2019.

131 AARP Global Council on Brain Health (2019). *The Real Deal on Brain Health Supplements.*

132 AARP Global Council on Brain Health (2019). *The Real Deal on Brain Health Supplements.*

133 Nutaitis, A. C., Tharwani, S. D., Serra, M. C., et al. (2019). "Diet as a risk factor for cognitive decline in African Americans and Caucasians with a parental history of Alzheimer's disease: A cross-sectional pilot study dietary patterns." *Journal of Prevention of Alzheimer's Disease* 6(1): 50–55.

134 Dohrmann, D. D., Putnik, P., Bursać Kovačević, D., Simal-Gandara, J., Lorenzo, J. M., Barba, F. J. (2019). "Japanese, Mediterranean and Argentinean diets and their potential roles in neurodegenerative diseases." *Food Research International* 120: 464–77.

135 McGrattan, A. M., McGuinness, B., McKinley, M. C., et al. (2019). "Diet and inflammation in cognitive ageing and Alzheimer's disease." *Current Nutrition Reports* 8(2): 53–65.

136 Abbatecola, A. M., Russo, M., & Barbieri, M. (2018). "Dietary patterns and cognition in older persons." *Current Opinion in Clinical Nutrition & Metabolic Care* 21(1): 10–13.

137 Hill et al., "Diet and biomarkers of Alzheimer's disease," 45–52.

138 Samadi, M., Moradi, S., Moradinazar, M., Mostafai, R., & Pasdar, Y. (2019). "Dietary pattern in relation to the risk of Alzheimer's disease: A systematic review." *Neurological Sciences,* June 25, 2019. doi: 10.1007/s10072-019-03976-3. [Epub ahead of print]

139 Solfrizzi et al., "Relationships of dietary patterns, foods, and micro- and macronutrients," 815–49.

140 Chen et al. "Dietary patterns and cognitive health in older adults," 583–619; Klímová & Vališ, "Nutritional Interventions," pii: E905; Solfrizzi et al., "Relationships of dietary patterns, foods, and micro- and macronutrients," 815–49.

Chapter 6 • Engage and Learn

141 Verghese, J., Le Valley, A., Derby, C. K., et al. (2006). "Leisure activities and the risk of amnesic mild cognitive impairment in the elderly." *Neurology* 66: 821–27.

142 Stern, C., & Munn, Z. (2010). "Cognitive leisure activities and their role in preventing dementia: A systematic review." *International Journal of Evidence-Based Healthcare* 8(1): 2–17.

143 Roberts, R. O., Cha, R. H., Mielke, M. M., et al. (2015). "Risk and protective factors for cognitive impairment in persons aged 85 years and older." *Neurology* 84(18): 1854–61.

144 Katzman, R. (1993). "Education and the prevalence of dementia and Alzheimer's disease. *Neurology* 43(1): 13–20.

145 Wilson, R. S., Bennett, D. A., Bienias, J. L., et al. (2002). "Cognitive activity and incident AD in a population-based sample of older persons." *Neurology* 59(12): 1910–14.

146 Wilson, R. S, Scherr, P. A., Schneider, J. A., Tang, Y., & Bennett, D. A. (2007). "Relation of cognitive activity to risk of developing Alzheimer disease." *Neurology* 69(20): 1911–20.

147 Valenzuela, M. J., & Sachdev, P. (2006). "Brain reserve and dementia: A systematic review." *Psychological Medicine* 36(4): 441–54.

148 Verghese, J., Le Valley, A., Derby, C., et al. (2006). "Leisure activities and the risk of amnestic mild cognitive impairment in the elderly." *Neurology* 66(6): 821–27.

149 Yates, L. A., Ziser, S., Spector, A., & Orrell, M. (2016). "Cognitive leisure activities and future risk of cognitive impairment and dementia: Systematic review and meta-analysis." *International Psychogeriatrics* 28(11): 1791–1806.

150 Najar, J., Östling, S., Gudmundsson, P., et al. (2019). "Cognitive and physical activity and dementia: A 44-year longitudinal population study of women." *Neurology* 92(12): e1322–30.

151 Wilson, R. D., Scherr, P. A., Schneider, J. A., Tang, Y., & Bennett, D. A. (2007). "Relation of cognitive activity to risk of developing Alzheimer disease." *Neurology* 69(20): 1911–20; Negash, S., Wilson, R. S., Leurgans, S. E., et al. (2013). "Resilient brain aging: Characterization of discordance between Alzheimer's disease pathology

and cognition." *Current Alzheimer Research* 10(8): 844–51; Wilson, R. S., Segawa, E., Boyle, P. A., & Bennet, D. A. (2012). "Influence of late-life cognitive activity on cognitive health." *Neurology* 78(15): 1123–29.

152 Verghese, J., Lipton, R. B., Katz, M. J., et al. (2003). "Leisure activities and the risk of dementia in the elderly." *New England Journal of Medicine* 348(25): 2508–16.

153 Hall, C. B., Lipton, R. B., Sliwinski, M., Katz, M. J., Derby, C. A., & Verghese, J. (2009). "Cognitive activities delay onset of memory decline in persons who develop dementia." *Neurology* 73(5): 356–61.

154 Kelly, M. E., Duff, H., Kelly, S., et al. (2017). "The impact of social activities, social networks, social support and social relationships on the cognitive functioning of healthy older adults: A systematic review." *Systematic Reviews* 6(1): 259; La Fleur, C. G., & Salthouse, T. A. (2017). "Which aspects of social support are associated with which cognitive abilities for which people?" *Journals of Gerontology. Series B, Psychological Sciences and Social Sciences* 72(6): 1006–16.

155 Janevic, M. R., Janz, N. K., Dodge, J. A., Wang, Y., Lin, X., & Clark, N. M. (2004). "Longitudinal effects of social support on the health and functioning of older women with heart disease." *International Journal of Aging and Human Development* 59(2): 153–75.

156 Clare, L., & Woods, R. T. (2004). "Cognitive training and cognitive rehabilitation for people with early-stage Alzheimer's disease: A review." *Neuropsychological Rehabilitation* 14(4): 385–401.

157 Clare & Woods, "Cognitive training and cognitive rehabilitation," 385–401.

158 Max Planck Institute for Human Development and Stanford Center on Longevity. *A Consensus on the Brain Training Industry from the Scientific Community*, 2014. http://longevity.stanford.edu/a-consensus-on-the-brain-training-industry-from-the-scientific-community-2/. Retrieved 8/3/2019.

159 Simons, D. J., Boot, W. R., Charness, S. E., et al. (2016). "Do 'brain-training' programs work?" *Psychological Science in the Public Interest* 17(3): 103.

160 Willis, S. L., Tennstedt, S. L., Marsiske, M., et al. (2006). "Long-term effects of cognitive training on everyday functional outcomes in older adults." *JAMA* 296(23): 2805–14.

161 Edwards, J. D., Xu, H., Clark, D., Ross, L. A., & Unverzagt, F. W. (2016). "The ACTIVE study: What we have learned and what is next? Cognitive training reduces incident dementia across ten years." *Alzheimer's & Dementia* 12(7): P212.

162 Edwards et al., "The ACTIVE study," P212.

163 Shao, Y., Mang, J., Li, P. L., Wang, J., Deng, T., & Xu, Z. X. (2015). "Computer-based cognitive programs for improvement of memory, processing speed and executive function during age-related cognitive decline: A meta-analysis." *PLOS One* 10(6): e0130831.

164 Lampit, A., Hallock, H., & Valenzuela, M. (2014). "Computerized cognitive training in cognitively healthy older adults: A systematic review and meta-analysis of effect modifiers." *PLOS Med* 11(11): e1001756.

165 Edwards, J. D., Fausto, B. A., Tetlow, A. M., Corona, R. T., & Valdés, E. G. (2018). "Systematic review and meta-analyses of useful field of view cognitive training." *Neuroscience & Biobehavioral Reviews* 84: 72–91.

166 Smith, G. E., Housen, P., Yaffe, K., et al. (2009). "A cognitive training program based on principles of brain plasticity: Results from the Improvement in Memory with

Plasticity-Based Adaptive Cognitive Training (IMPACT) Study." *Journal of the American Geriatrics Society* 57(4): 594–603.

167 Corbett, A., Owen, A., Hampshire, A., et al. (2015). "The effect of an online cognitive training package in healthy older adults: An online randomized controlled trial." *Journal of the American Medical Directors Association* 16(11): 990–97.

168 Institute of Medicine of the National Academies. *Cognitive Aging: Progress in Understanding and Opportunities for Action*, 2015. https://www.nap.edu/read/21693/chapter/1.

169 Institute of Medicine of the National Academies, *Cognitive Aging*.

Chapter 7 • Lower Stress and Boost Well-Being

170 Aggarwal, N. T., Wilson, R. S., Beck, T. L., et al. (2014). "Perceived stress and change in cognitive function among adults aged 65 and older." *Psychosomatic Medicine* 6(1): 80–85.

171 Tschanz, J. T., Pfister, R., Wanzek, J., et al. (2013). "Stressful life events and cognitive decline in late life: Moderation by education and age: The Cache County Study." *International Journal of Geriatric Psychiatry* 28(8): 821–30.

172 Korten, N. C. M., Comijs, H. C., Penninx, B. W., et al. (2017). "Perceived stress and cognitive function in older adults: Which aspect of perceived stress is important?" *International Journal of Geriatric Psychiatry* 21(4): 439–45.

173 Katz, M. J., Derby, C. A., Wang, C., et al. (2016). "Influence of perceived stress on incident amnestic mild cognitive impairment: Results from the Einstein Aging Study." *Alzheimer's Disease & Associated Disorders* 30(2): 93–98.

174 Ishtiak-Ahmed, K., Garde, A. H., Gyntelberg, F., et al. (2019). "Perceived stress and dementia: Results from the Copenhagen City heart study." *Aging & Mental Health* 11: 1–9.

175 World Health Organization. *Depression and Other Common Mental Disorders: Global Health Estimates*, 2017. https://apps.who.int/iris/bitstream/handle/10665/254610/WHO-MSD-MER-2017.2-eng.pdf?sequence=1. Retrieved 8/3/2019.

176 Diniz, V. S., Butters, M. A., Albert, S. M., & Dew, M. A. (2013). "Late-life depression and risk of vascular dementia and Alzheimer's disease: Systematic review and meta-analysis of community-based cohort studies." *British Journal of Psychiatry* 202(5): 329–35.

177 Santabárbara, J., Sevil-Perez, A., Olaya, B., Gracia-García, P., & Lopez-Anton, R. (2019). "Clinically relevant late-life depression as risk factor of dementia: A systematic review and meta-analysis of prospective cohort studies." *Revista de neurologia* 68(12): 493–502; Leonard, B. E (2007). "Inflammation, depression and dementia: Are they connected?" *Neurochemical Research* 32(10): 1749–56.

178 Sugarman, M. A., Alosco, M. L., Tripodis, Y., Steinberg, E. G., & Stern, R. A. (2018). "Neuropsychiatric symptoms and the diagnostic stability of mild cognitive impairment." *Journal of Alzheimer's Disease* 62(4): 1841–55.

179 Taylor, W. D., McQuoid, D. R., Payne, M. E., Zannas, A. S., MacFall, J. R., & Steffens, D. C. (2014). "Hippocampus atrophy and the longitudinal course of late-life depression." *American Journal of Geriatric Psychiatry* 22(12): 1504–12.

180 Edwards, G. A., III, Gamez, N., Escobedo, G., Jr., Calderon, O., & Moreno-Gonzalez, I. (2019). "Modifiable risk factors for Alzheimer's disease." *Frontiers in Aging Neuroscience* 11: 146; Ross, J. A., Gliebus, G., & Van Bockstaele, E. J. (2018). "Stress induced neural reorganization: A conceptual framework linking depression

and Alzheimer's disease." *Progress in Neuropsychopharmacology & Biological Psychiatry* 85: 136–51.

181 Leonard, "Inflammation, depression and dementia," 1749–56.

182 Barnes & Yaffe, "The projected impact of risk factor reduction on Alzheimer's, 819–28.

183 Sugarman, M. A., Alosco, M. L., Tripodis, Y., Steinberg, E. G., & Stern, R. A. (2018). "Neuropsychiatric symptoms and the diagnostic stability of mild cognitive impairment." *Journal of Alzheimer's Disease* 62(4): 1841–55.

184 Butters, M. A., Becker, J. T., Nebes, R. D., et al. (2000). "Changes in cognitive functioning following treatment of late-life depression." *American Journal of Psychiatry* 157: 1949–54; Gallassi, R., Di Sarro, R., Morreale, A., & Amore, M. (2006). "Memory impairment in patients with late-onset major depression: The effect of antidepressant therapy." *Journal of Affective Disorders* 91: 243–50.

185 Diniz et al., "Late-life depression and risk of vascular dementia," 329–35.

186 Reynolds, C. F., III, Cuijpers, P., Patel, V., et al. (2012). "Early intervention to reduce the global health and economic burden of major depression in older adults." *Annual Review of Public Health* 33: 123–35; Cuijpers, P., Berking, M., Andersson, G., Quigley, L., Kleiboer, A., & Dobson, K. S. (2013). "A meta-analysis of cognitive-behavioural therapy for adult depression, alone and in comparison with other treatments." *Canadian Journal of Psychiatry* 58(7): 376–85.

187 Reynolds III et al. "Early intervention to reduce the global health," 123–35.

188 Llewellyn, D. A., Lang, I. A., Langa, K. M., & Hupper, F. A. (2008). "Cognitive function and psychological well-being: Findings from a population-based cohort." *Age and Ageing* 37(6): 685–89; Allerhand, M., Gale, C. R., & Deary, I. J. (2014). "The dynamic relationship between cognitive function and positive well-being in older people: A prospective study using the English Longitudinal Study of Aging." *Psychology and Aging* 29(2): 306–18.

189 Allerhand, Gale, & Deary, "The dynamic relationship between cognitive function," 306–18.

190 Wegner, M., Helmich, I., Machado, S., Nardi, A. E., Arias-Carrion, O., & Budde, H. (2014). "Effects of exercise on anxiety and depression disorders: Review of meta-analyses and neurobiological mechanisms." *CNS & Neurological Disorders—Drug Targets* 13(6): 1002–14.

191 Kvam, S., Kleppe, C. L., Nordhus, I. H., & Hovland, A. (2016). "Exercise as a treatment for depression: A meta-analysis." *Journal of Affective Disorders* 202: 67–86; Gujral, S., Aizenstein, H., Reynolds, C. F., et al. (2019). "Exercise for depression: A feasibility trial exploring neural mechanisms." *American Journal of Geriatric Psychiatry* pii: S1064–7481(19)30024-7.

192 Zhang, Z., & Chen, W. (2019). "A systematic review of the relationship between physical activity and happiness." *Journal of Happiness Studies* 20(4): 1305–22.

193 Lenze, E. J., Hickman, S., Hershey, T., et al. (2014). "Mindfulness-based stress reduction for older adults with worry symptoms and co-occurring cognitive dysfunction." *International Journal of Geriatric Psychiatry* 29(10): 991–1000; Wetherell, J. L., Hershey, T., Hickman, S., et al. (2017). "Mindfulness-based stress reduction for older adults with stress disorders and neurocognitive difficulties: A randomized controlled trial. *Journal of Clinical Psychiatry* 78(7): e734–43.

194 Wetherell et al., "Mindfulness-based stress reduction for older adults with stress disorders," e734–43; Parmentier, F. B. R., García-Toro, M., García-Campayo, J., et

al. (2019). "Mindfulness and symptoms of depression and anxiety in the general population: The mediating roles of worry, rumination, reappraisal and suppression." *Frontiers in Psychology* 10: 506.

195 Lenze et al., "Mindfulness-based stress reduction for older adults with worry symptoms," 991–1000.

196 Lardone, A., Liparoti, M., Sorrento, P., et al. (2018). "Mindfulness meditation is related to long-lasting changes in hippocampal functional topology during resting state: A magnetoencephalography study." *Neural Plasticity* 5340717. doi: 10.1155/2018/5340717

197 Hölzel, B. K., Carmody, J., & Vangel, M. (2011). "Mindfulness practice leads to increases in regional brain gray matter density." *Psychiatry Research* 191(1): 36–43.

198 Marciniak, R., Sheardova, K., Cermáková, P., et al. (2014). "Effect of meditation on cognitive functions in context of aging and neurodegenerative diseases." *Frontiers in Behavioral Neuroscience* 8: 17.

199 Gard, T., Hölzel, B. K., & Lazar, S. W. (2014). "The potential effects of meditation on age-related cognitive decline: A systematic review." *Annals of the New York Academy of Sciences* 1307: 89–103.

200 Innes, K. E., Selfe, T. K., Brundage, K., et al. (2018). "Effects of meditation and music-listening on blood biomarkers of cellular aging and Alzheimer's disease in adults with subjective cognitive decline: An exploratory randomized clinical trial." *Journal of Alzheimer's Disease* 66(3): 947–70.

201 Innes et al., "Effects of meditation and music-listening," 947–70; Chaix, R., Alvarez-López, M. J., Fagny, M., et al. (2017). "Epigenetic clock analysis in long-term meditators." *Psychoneuroendocrinology* 85: 210–14.

202 Chaix et al., "Epigenetic clock analysis," 210–14.

203 Greenberg, J., Romero, V. L., Elkin-Frankson, S., et al. (2019). "Reduced interference in working memory following mindfulness training is associated with increases in hippocampal volume." *Brain Imaging and Behavior* 13(2): 366–76.

204 Bishop, S. R., Lau, M., Shapiro, S., et al. (2004). "Mindfulness: A proposed operational definition." *Clinical Psychology: Science and Practice* 11: 23–41.

205 Hosseini, S., Chaurasia, A., & Oremus, M. (2019). "The effect of religion and spirituality on cognitive function: A systematic review." *Gerontologist* 59(2): e76–85.

206 Wu, G., Feder, A., Cohen, H., Kim, J. J., Carney, D. S., & Mathé, A. A. (2013). "Understanding resilience." *Frontiers in Behavioral Neuroscience* 7: 10.

207 Wu et al., "Understanding resilience," 10.

208 Lamond, A. J., Depp, C. A., Allison, M., et al. (2008). "Measurement and predictors of resilience among community-dwelling older women." *Journal of Psychiatric Research* 43(2): 148–54.

Chapter 8 • Sleep for Better Brain Power

209 AARP, *2015 Survey on Brain Health.*

210 Sara, S. J. (2017). "Sleep to remember." *Journal of Neuroscience* 37(3): 457–63; Ackermann, S., & Rasch, B. (2014). "Differential effects of non-REM and REM sleep on memory consolidation?" *Current Neurology and Neuroscience Reports* 14(2): 430.

211 Sara, "Sleep to remember," 457–63.

212 Sara, "Sleep to remember," 457–63; Peter-Derex, L. (2019). "Sleep and memory consolidation." *Neurophysiologie clinique* 49(3): 197–98.

213 Sara, "Sleep to remember," 457–63.

214 Schapiro, A. C., Reid, A. G., Morgan, A., Manoach, D. S., Verfaellie, M., & Stickgold, R. (2019). "The hippocampus is necessary for the consolidation of a task that does not require the hippocampus for initial learning." *Hippocampus* doi: 10.1002/hipo.23101. [Epub ahead of print]

215 Tsapanou, A., Vlachos, G. S., Cosentino, S., et al. (2018). "Sleep and subjective cognitive decline in cognitively healthy elderly: Results from two cohorts." *Journal of Sleep Research.* doi: 10.1111/jsr.12759. [Epub ahead of print]; Ramos, A. R., Gardener, H., Rundek, T., et. al. (2016). "Sleep disturbances and cognitive decline in the Northern Manhattan Study." *Neurology* 87(14): 1511–16.

216 Lo, J. C., Groeger, J. A., Cheng, G. H., Dijk, D. J., & Chee, M. W. (2016). "Self-reported sleep duration and cognitive performance in older adults: A systematic review and meta-analysis." *Sleep Medicine* 17: 87–98.

217 Lo, J. C. et al., "Self-reported sleep duration and cognitive performance," 87–98.

218 Low, D. V., Wu, M. N., & Spira, A. P. (2019). "Sleep duration and cognition in a nationally representative sample of U.S. older adults." *American Journal of Geriatric Psychiatry.* pii: S1064-7481(19)30426-9.

219 Yaffe, K., Falvey, C. M., & Hoang, T. (2014). "Connections between sleep and cognition in older adults." *Lancet Neurology* 13: 1017–28.

220 Bubu, O. M., Brannick, M., Mortimer, J., et al. (2017). "Sleep, cognitive impairment, and Alzheimer's disease: A systematic review and meta-analysis." *Sleep* 40(1). doi: 10.1093/sleep/zsw032.

221 Spira & Gottesman, "Sleep disturbance," 529–31.

222 Senaratna, C. V., Perret, J. L., Lodge, C. J., et al. (2017). "Prevalence of obstructive sleep apnea in the general population: A systematic review." *Sleep Medicine Reviews* 34: 70–81.

223 Roth, T. (2007). "Insomnia: Definition, prevalence, etiology, and consequences." *Journal of Clinical Sleep Medicine* 3(5 Suppl): S7–10.

224 Spira & Gottesman, "Sleep disturbance," 529–31; Spira, A. P. (2015). "Being mindful of later-life sleep quality and its potential role in prevention." *JAMA Internal Medicine* 175(4): 502–03.

225 Yang, P. Y., Ho, K. H., Chen, H. C., & Chien, M. Y. (2012). "Exercise training improves sleep quality in middle-aged and older adults with sleep problems: A systematic review." *Journal of Physiotherapy* 58(3): 157–63.

226 Chen, L. J., Fox, K. R., Ku, P. W., & Chang, Y. W. (2016). "Effects of aquatic exercise on sleep in older adults with mild sleep impairment: A randomized controlled trial." *International Journal of Behavioral Medicine* 23(4): 501–06.

227 Chen, L. J., Stevinson, C., Fang, S. H., Taun, C. Y., & Ku, P. W. (2019). "Effects of an acute bout of light-intensity walking on sleep in older women with sleep impairment: A randomized controlled trial." *Journal of Clinical Sleep Medicine* 15(4): 581–86.

228 Reid, K. J., Baron, K. G., Lu, B., Naylor, E., Wolfe, L., & Zee, P. C. (2010). "Aerobic exercise improves self-reported sleep and quality of life in older adults with insomnia." *Sleep Medicine* 11(9): 934–40.

229 Black, D. S., O'Reilly, G. A., Olmstead, R., Green, E. C., & Irwin, M. R. (2015). "Mindfulness meditation and improvement in sleep quality and daytime impairment among older adults with sleep disturbances: A randomized clinical trial." *JAMA Internal Medicine* 175(4): 494–501.

230 Spira, "Being mindful of later-life sleep quality," 502–3.

231 Fitzgerald, T., & Vietri, J. (2015). "Residual effects of sleep medications are commonly reported and associated with impaired patient-reported outcomes among

insomnia patients in the United States." *Sleep Disorders 2015:* 607148. doi: 10.1155/2015/607148.

232 Irish, L. A., Kline, C. E., Gunn, H. E., Buysse, D. J., & Hall, M. H. (2015). "The role of sleep hygiene in promoting public health: A review of empirical evidence." *Sleep Medicine Reviews* 22: 23–36; Chung, K. F., Lee, C. T., Yeung, W. F., Chan, M. S., Chung, E. W., & Lin, W. L. (2018). "Sleep hygiene education as a treatment of insomnia: A systematic review and meta-analysis." *Family Practice* 35(4): 365–75.

233 Zimmerman, M. E., Kim, M. B., Hale, C., Westwood, A. J., Brickman, A. M., & Shechter, A. (2019). "Neuropsychological function response to nocturnal blue light blockage in individuals with symptoms of insomnia: A pilot randomized controlled study." *Journal of the International Neuropsychological Society* 20: 1–10.

234 Roehrs, T., Shambroom, J., & Roth, T. (2013). "Caffeine effects on sleep taken 0, 3, or 6 hours before going to bed." *Journal of Clinical Sleep Medicine* 9(11): 1195–1200.

235 Ebrahim, I. O., Shapiro, C. M., Williams, A. J., & Fenwick, P. B. (2013). "Alcohol and sleep. I: Effects on normal sleep." *Alcoholism: Clinical and Experimental Research* 7(4): 539–49.

236 Li, M. J., Kechter, A., Olmstead, R. E., Irwin, M. R., & Black, D. S. (2018). "Sleep and mood in older adults: Coinciding changes in insomnia and depression symptoms." *International Psychogeriatrics* 30(3): 431–35.

Brain Health Expert Contributors

Chapter 1: Dr. Sandra Weintraub—SuperAgers

Dr. Sandra Weintraub is a professor of psychiatry, behavioral sciences, and neurology at Northwestern University Feinberg School of Medicine. Dr. Weintraub and her colleagues Drs. Marsel Mesulam, Emily Rogalski, and Changiz Geula created the now global concept of SuperAgers. Research on SuperAgers has provided fascinating—and sometimes surprising—insights about this rare group of individuals.

Chapter 3: Dr. Marwan Sabbagh—Changing Your Mind-Set

Dr. Marwan Sabbagh is a board-certified neurologist, director of the Cleveland Clinic Lou Ruvo Center for Brain Health, and clinical professor in the Department of Neurology at the University of Nevada, Las Vegas. Dr. Sabbagh has authored and co-authored almost 300 medical and scientific articles on Alzheimer's research. He is the author of *The Alzheimer's Answer: Reduce Your Risk and Keep Your Brain Healthy* and a co-author of *The Alzheimer's Prevention Cookbook: 100 Recipes to Boost Brain Health* and *Fighting for My Life: How to Thrive in the Shadow of Alzheimer's*.

Chapter 4: Dr. Kirk Erickson—Exercise, Cognitive Functioning, and Brain Health

Dr. Kirk Erickson is a professor in the Department of Psychology at the University of Pittsburgh's Center for the Neural Basis of Cognition. He is a fellow of the Academy of Behavioral Medicine Research and the recipient of the University of Pittsburgh Chancellor's Distinguished Research Award. He has received funding from the National Institutes of Health (NIH) for several years and has authored and co-authored approximately 175 medical and scientific articles and 14 book chapters on exercise and cognition. He is the principal investigator in several ongoing studies, including a five-year randomized trial examining exercise and cognition.

Chapter 5: Dr. Martha Clare Morris—The MIND Diet

Dr. Martha Clare Morris is professor of epidemiology, the director of the Rush Institute for Healthy Aging, and assistant provost of community research at Rush University Medical Center in Chicago. She has more than 20 years of experience studying the relationship between nutrition and the development of Alzheimer's disease and is the lead creator of the MIND diet for healthy brain aging. Dr. Morris has a long history of funding from the National Institutes of Health (NIH) and has examined dietary risk factors of Alzheimer's disease among 10,000 African Americans and white Americans in the Chicago Health and Aging Project and over 1,000 participants in the Memory and Aging Project. Dr. Morris is the author of *Diet for the MIND: The Latest Science on What to Eat to Prevent Alzheimer's and Cognitive Decline.*

Chapter 6: Dr. Yaakov Stern—Cognitive Reserve, Aging, and Alzheimer's

Dr. Yaakov Stern is a professor of neuropsychology at the Taub Institute for Research on Alzheimer's Disease and the Aging Brain and chief of the Cognitive Neuroscience Division in the Department of Neurology at Columbia University Medical Center in New York City. He is internationally recognized for his research in cognitive reserve, aging, and Alzheimer's disease and is currently investigating the neural basis of cognitive reserve.

Chapter 7: Dr. Jonathan Greenberg—Mindfulness, Brain Health, and Well-Being

Dr. Greenberg is a clinical and research fellow in the Integrated Brain Health Clinical and Research Program of the Department of Psychiatry in Massachusetts General Hospital and Harvard Medical School. He researches the impact of mind-body and mindfulness training on cognitive, emotional, and physical function among individuals with chronic pain, injuries, and depression, among other conditions.

Chapter 8: Dr. Brendan Lucey—Sleep, Alzheimer's, and Brain Health

Brendan Lucey, MD, is the director of sleep medicine and assistant professor of neurology at Washington University School of Medicine. He is board-certified in neurology and sleep medicine and has authored many medical and scientific articles on sleep and Alzheimer's. His research on the relationship between sleep deprivation and increased levels of beta-amyloid and tau—proteins involved in Alzheimer's—has received widespread recognition for its importance.

Appendix II: Dr. Melanie Chandler—Treatment of Mild Cognitive Impairment

Dr. Melanie Chandler is the Director of HABIT at the Mayo Clinic in Florida. HABIT (Healthy Action to Benefit Independence & Thinking) includes memory training, cognitive exercise, yoga, wellness education, and support groups for individuals with MCI and their care partners. She and her colleagues have published research showing that HABIT participants report improved daily functioning, mood, and quality of life, among other positive changes, after completing the program. She is currently conducting a clinical trial on HABIT and hoping to expand the number of locations in which the program is offered.

Index

AARP GCBH report, 93–94

Accelerated aging, 10, 11–14, 45, 51, 53, 54, 56, 83, 94, 110. *See also* brain health trajectories, Memory

Accountability partners, 30, 40, 206–7

ACTIVE study, 118–19

Aducanumab (drug), 2

Age, as foundational factor, 45

Aging
    accelerated, 10, 11–14, 45, 51, 53, 54, 56, 83, 94, 110
    brain, optimal, 26, 28, 42, 45, 53, 56
    cellular, meditation and, 133, 135; Telomeres and, 32; physical activity and, 71, 133
    normal, 3, 10, 11, 12, 45, 56
    pathways, 23–24
    upside of, 23

Alcohol, 2, 47, 48, 59, 82, 90, 94, 96, 158, 161

Alzheimer, Dr. Alois, 12

Alzheimer's. *See also individual topics*
    autosomal-dominant, 32
    beginning of, 13
    cellular abnormalities, 18, 21, 22, 98–99
    compensation and, 112
    confusion around, 9–10
    defined, 12
    as "defining disease for baby boomers," 9
    depression and, 131–32, 133
    diet link, 98–99
    drugs, failure of, 2
    fear of, 9
    future brain health improvement and, 2
    genetic risk factors, 27; *see also* Genetic risk for Alzheimer's
    lifestyle factors and, 2, 3, 9
    MIND diet and, 84
    misconceptions, 3
    no direct cause for, 10
    predicators, Nun Study and, 20–21

questions about, 8–9

research, 3

risk, as increasing with age, 12–13

as "silent," 27

sleep and, 153–59, 165

slow-wave sleep and, 156

statistics, 2, 9

stress and, 129, 149

use of term, this book, xv

Alzheimer's-related cellular changes
    Alzheimer's symptoms and, 22
    compensating for, 112
    diet and, 98–99
    lifestyle factors and, 2–3
    SuperAgers and, 24

Alzheimer's risk factors
    brain-healthy diet and, 85
    family history and, 3, 46
    foundational factors and, 45–47
    health-related, 47
    lifestyle, 47–48
    vascular, 47

Alzheimer's symptoms, 2, 13, 22

Alzheimer's treatment
    about, 13–14
    aerobic exercise and, 13–14
    MIND-AD and, 14
    sleep and, 156–57

Amy, age 44 (role model), 169–72

Amyloid beta. *See* Beta-amyloid

Anticholinergic medications, 47

APOE-e4, FINGER study and, 31

Artistic engagement, cognitive reserve and, 114–15

Autobiographical memory, 140

Autosomal-dominant Alzheimer's, 32

Berries, 83, 84, 87, 91

Beta-amyloid, 12, 32, 60, 71, 97, 98, 134–35, 154, 155, 156, 157, 259

Bilingualism, 46
"Boost Your Brain" presentations, 4
Brain blips
    defined, 8
    forgetting new information, 123
    forgetting new names, 120–21
    misplacing objects, 121–22
    Pause-Link-Rehearse and, 120–23, 128
    quiz, 16
    tips for, 120–25
    word-finding difficulties, 124–25
Brain-derived neurotrophic factor, 60–61, 62
Brain function
    Alzheimer's and, 12
    exercise and, 71
    healthy diet and, 98, 106
    improving, 10, 93
    optimizing, xi–xii, xv
Brain games. See also computerized
        cognitive training
    benefits of, 128
    cognitive functioning and, 117–20
    cognitive reserve and, 114–15
    as enhancement technique, 117
Brain health. See also healthy brain habits
    alcohol and, 47, 48, 59, 82, 90, 94, 96,
        158, 161
    building, into busy life, 43–44
    exercise and, 60–61, 64
    heart health and, xi
    improving, 2
    lifestyle factors and, 1, 3
    MIND diet and, 84
    misconceptions, 3
    most helpful interventions, 42
    Psychology Today blog on, xii
    questions about, 8–9
    science of, 1, 3, 4
    strategies, in practice, 3
    three-path choice regarding, 51
Brain health highlights (role models)
    Amy, age 44, 172
    Bill, age 93, 195–96
    Byung, age 72, 183–84
    Caroline, age 100, 199–200
    Edna, age 103, 203–4
    Jan, age 62, 179–80
    Otto, age 91, 191–92
    Sue, age 83, 186–87

Virgil, age 53, 175–76
Brain Health Myth Busters, 21, 27
Brain health supplements, 42, 43, 92–94,
        105
Brain health trajectories
    accelerated aging, 10, 11–14, 45, 51, 53,
        54, 56, 83, 94, 110
    determination of, 27
    enhancing, 32
    graph, 10
    High-Octane Brain, 10, 18–26
    lifestyle factors and, 47–48
    Navigational Forces and, 45–48
    normal aging, 10, 11, 45, 56
    shifting, 44–45
Brains, xii, 1, 11
Brain volume, exercise and, 60
Bronx Aging Study, 110
Byung, age 72 (role model), 180–84

Cellular and metabolic changes, exercise
        and, 71
Chandler, Dr. Melanie, 231–39
Chicago Health and Aging Project, 108
Coffee and tea, 90
Cognitive Activity Scale (CAS), 109, 128
Cognitive Behavioral Therapy for Insomnia
        (CBTI), 157, 159
Cognitive compensation tools
    about, 116, 128
    for brain blips, 120–25
    name of someone you just met, 121
    new information, 123
    object placement, 121
    word finding, 124–25
Cognitive engagement
    about, 107
    benefits of, 107
    cognitive reserve and, 108–9
    measurement of, 109
    mild cognitive impairment (MCI) and,
        108
    work and, 113–14
Cognitive enhancement tools, 116–17
Cognitive functioning
    cognitive stimulation techniques and,
        116–17
    cognitive training and brain games and,
        117–20

Cognitive functioning (*continued*)
   enhancement strategies, 116–17
   mindfulness and, 139–40, 141
   mood connection, 149
   sleep and, 153–59, 165
   stress and, 131
   tools for enhancing, 116–17
Cognitive reserve
   artistic engagement and, 114–15
   defined, 108, 111, 128
   importance of, 111
   increasing, 113
   low, brain function and, 111–12
   power of, 108–9, 128–29
   social engagement and, 114–15
   stronger, activities linked to, 115
Cognitive stimulation, 116–17
Cognitive training, 116–17. *See also* brain
   games
Compensation, 112
Computerized cognitive training (CCT).
   See also brain games
   about, 117–18
   ACTIVE, 118–19
   benefits of, 118
   defined, 117
   effectiveness, 119–20
   in IMPACT trial, 119
   issues, 119–20
   Useful Field of View, 119
Cortisol, 134
CPAP (continuous positive airway pressure),
   158
Crossword puzzles, 3, 8, 109, 115, 116, 128
Csikszentmihalyi, Dr. Mihaly, 144

DASH diet, 82, 83, 84, 85, 89, 99, 102, 105
Dementia. *See also* Alzheimer's
   defined, 12
   exercise and, 59
   mild cognitive impairment (MCI)
      versus, 15
   normal aging and, 12
   risks of, 9, 59
   stress and, 131
Depression
   Alzheimer's and, 131–32, 133
   mindfulness and, 134–35, 141
   physical exercise and, 133–34

   reduction in, 133
   stress and, 131, 132, 149
   symptoms, 131
   treatment of, 132–33
Diet. *See also* MIND diet
   Alzheimer's link, 98–99
   brain health, one size not fitting all, 95
   brain-healthy, 85
   cellular abnormalities and, 98–99
   culturally specific, 91, 105
   DASH, 82, 83, 84, 85, 89, 99, 102, 105
   healthy, benefits of, 98, 106
   Mediterranean, 82, 83, 84, 85, 89, 99,
      102, 105
   misconceptions, brain health and,
      89–90
   nutrients and, 96–98, 106
   successful changes to, 92
   Takeaways, 105–6
DNA methylation, 42

Educational level, 46, 110, 112
Engage and learn
   about, 107
   brain blip tips and, 120–25
   cognitive engagement, 109–16
   cognitive functioning strategies, 116–17
   cognitive reserve and, 108–9, 111–12,
      113, 114–15
   computerized cognitive training (CCT)
      and, 117
   High-Octane Action Plan, 125–26
   Takeaways, 128
Epigenetics
   defined, 1, 32, 42
   gene expression, altering and, 45, 55
   High-Octane Brain and, 32–33
   power of, 42–43, 44–48
Epilepsy (seizures), 47
Erickson, Dr. Kirk, 61–62, 64–70
EXCELS Method
   acronym, 49, 53
   defined, 49, 56
   engage and learn, 126
   High-Octane Tracker and, 214, 215
   one step impacting others and, 149
   steps, 49, 50
   steps, basis of, 49–50
   steps, following, 51, 52

Exercise. *See also* lifestyle factors
  activity selection, 65, 72–73
  acute bouts of, brain performance and, 67
  alternative forms of, 68
  as Alzheimer's treatment, 13–14
  amount, any as beneficial, 66, 76–77, 79
  amplified High-Octane Brain benefits, 135
  autosomal-dominant Alzheimer's and, 32
  BDNF and, 62
  beginning later in life, 67–68
  as beneficial brain health intervention, 42
  Bonus Benefits of, 60, 70–71, 79
  brain health and, 60–61, 64
  as depression intervention, 133–34
  each person as different and, 66–67
  in early life, 68
  habit, how to begin, 64–65
  happiness link, 134
  helping to maintain, 65
  High-Octane Action Plan, 70
  High-Octane Tracker, 74–75, 78
  hippocampal growth and, 62, 63, 76
  Immediate Boost, 73–74, 77
  intensity, any as beneficial, 73
  as lasting habit, 79
  length of time per week, 66, 76, 79
  midlife, dementia and, 59
  mild cognitive impairment (MCI) and, 231, 235
  mindfulness and, 68
  neurogenesis and, xi
  as neurogenesis trigger, xi
  neuroplasticity and, 60
  as not a magic bullet, 69
  optimal amount of, 65–66
  organ systems and, 64
  positive benefits of, 70
  sleep and, 159, 161
  studies of dementia and, 58–60
  Swedish women study, 58–59
  Takeaways, 79–80
  top limit of, 67
  as X-factor, 49, 70, 79–80
"Exergaming," 68
EXERT clinical trial, 15

Fabulous Four, 19–22, 107
Family history for Alzheimer's, 3, 45–46
Fats, saturated and trans, 88
FINGER study, 31–32, 40, 95
Five-step tracking system. *See* High-Octane Tracker
Flow, 144
Foods, brain-healthy, 83, 86–87, 99–102. *See also* MIND diet
Forgetfulness, 16–17
Foundational factors, 33, 45–47

Games
  brain, 117–20, 128
  cognitive reserve and, 115
  increased activity and, 68
  playing, engagement and, 107
Genetic risk for Alzheimer's, 1, 5, 18, 21, 27, 31, 40
Genetics
  FINGER study and, 31–32
  as foundational factor, 45–46
  lifestyle choices and, 1, 9, 19
  SuperAgers and, 25

Greenberg, Dr. Jonathan, 135–44
Gut microbiome, 98

HABIT (Healthy Action to Benefit Independence & Thinking)
  defined, 15, 231
  development of, 232–33
  maintaining learned behaviors from, 237–38
  MCI benefits, 237
  meaningful benefit from, 239
  memory-related daily tasks, improvement in and, 234
  participant reports, 15, 231
  program expansion, 238
  support groups, 235–36, 237
  synergistic effect of components, 236
  those unable to access, 238–39
  yoga as physical intervention and, 234–35
Hall of Famers (role models), 188–204
Happiness, exercise, 134
Health-related factors, 47

Healthy brain habits. *See also* brain health
  adaptation to, 103–4
  cost of not integrating, 5
  hereditary risk of Alzheimer's and, 18–19
  making a choice for, 50–52
  Meredith and Lou integration of, 5–6
  putting into action, 43
  "rhythm," 53
High-Octane Action Plan
  about, 38–39
  activities that appeal to you, 125, 217
  beginning, 37, 40
  Bonus Benefits to physical activity, 70–71, 216
  as core of High-Octane Brain journey, 37
  creating, 29
  diet, 98–99
  engage and learn, 125
  exercise, 70–74
  how to use, 37, 214
  Ideal Future Self, 39, 216
  insights from High Octane Brain role models, 218
  joyful activities, 72–73, 217
  MIND diet, 99, 217
  positive stress management, 146, 217
  recommendations, 30
  resilience in action, 146, 218
  sleep improvement, 162, 218
  stress management, 145–46
  Three-Path Choice, 50–52, 216
  "Whys," your, 38–39, 216
High-Octane Brain
  approach, 5–6
  criterion-referenced definition, 26
  defined, 5, 18
  defining, 19, 33
  epigenetics and, 32–33
  experience of, 5
  lifestyle habits and, 28
  optimal brain aging and, 26
  outcomes, 5, 18, 26
  revolution, 8–28
High-Octane Brain class, 29–31, 37. *See also* Meredith and Lou
High-Octane Brain journey
  about, 6

  benefits of, 41
  High-Octane Action Plan and, 37
  ideal future self and, 38–39
  as journey of promise, 41
  preparing for, 29–31
  realization of choices in, 41
  social support for, 30, 40
  Whys, 38–39, 40, 52, 55, 126, 148, 206
High-Octane Brain path, 51, 53–55, 56
High-Octane Brain role models
  Amy, age 44, 169–72
  Bill, age 93, 193–96
  Byung, age 72, 180–84
  Caroline, age 100, 197–200
  Edna, age 103, 200–204
  "Hall of Famers," 184–87
  inspiration from, 169
  Jan, age 62, 176–80
  Otto, age 91, 189–92
  stories, about, xv, 168, 188
  "Success Squad," 168–87
  Sue, age 83, 184–87
  Virgil, age 53, 173–76
High-Octane Brain trajectory. *See also* brain health trajectories
  about, 18–19
  choosing, 52
  EXCELS Method and, 51
  Fabulous Four and, 19–22
  illustrated, 10
  outcomes, 18
  SuperAgers and, 22–26
High-Octane Tracker
  about, 3–4, 40
  "baseline" octane levels, 215
  in changing brain health habits, 33
  completion of, 215
  Consume Healthy Food scoring, 221, 223, 225, 228
  defined, 214
  diet: consume healthy food, 99–102
  diet: MIND diet, 100–101, 104
  diet: tips for success, 101–2
  engage and learn, 125–26
  EXCELS Method and, 214, 215
  exercise: illustrated, 78
  exercise: Tracking Phase 1, 74–75
  exercise: Tracking Phase 2, 75
  following, 29

gray columns, 215
how to use, 37, 214
Lower Stress and Boost Well-Being
    scoring, 226, 229
OCTANE, 77, 80
with a partner, 206
sleep, 163
Sleep for Better Brain Power scoring,
    230
Step 1, 219
Step 1–2, 220
Step 1–3, 222
Step 1–4, 224
Step 1–5, 224
stress management, 146–47
tips for using, 214–15
Hippocampal growth, 62, 63, 76, 135, 140
Hippocampus function, 13

Ideal Future Self
    exercise, 38–39
    High-Octane Brain path as leading
        to, 55
    Three Path Choice and, 54–55
Immediate Exercise Boost, 73–74, 77
IMPACT trial, 119
Information
    familiar, forgetting, 16–17
    new, forgetting, 123
    no longer relevant, decoupling, 140
Insomnia, 157, 159, 160, 161, 162. *See also*
    sleep
Inspiration, 19, 169, 206, 207
Instrumental activities of daily living
    (IADLs), 14–15

Jan, age 62 (role model), 176–80

Kabat-Zinn, Jon, 136, 142
Kotelko, Olga, 19–20

Languages, learning, 115
Learning. *See* engage and learn
Lifestyle factors. *See also* Navigational
    Forces; *specific factors*
    Alzheimer's and, 2, 3, 9
    brain health and, 1, 3
    brain health trajectory and, 47–48
    defined, 2

immediate benefits of, 41
as inflection point, 48
as navigational force, 47–48
positive feedback loops, 48
in successful agers, xii
Lucey, Dr. Brendan, 154–59

MAP study
    about, 81
    DASH diet and, 82, 84
    Mediterranean diet and, 82, 83, 84
    MIND diet, 83–85, 89–92
    participants in, 82
    results of, 84–85
Meditation
    benefits of, 134–35
    impact on hippocampal function and
        structure, 139
    mindfulness and, 136–37
    during work, 143
Mediterranean diet, 82, 83, 84, 85, 89, 99,
    102, 105
Memory
    autobiographical, 140
    optimizing, xv
    sleep and, 152–53
    working, 139, 140
Memory and Aging Project. *See* MAP study
Memory problems
    discussing with healthcare provider, 40
    forgetfulness and, 16–17
    mindfulness and, 140
    potential, warning signs of, 16–17
    quiz, 16
Memory Support System, 233–34
Meredith and Lou
    about, 34–36
    as accountability partners, 34, 207
    adjustments as they go, 147–48
    changes take hold, 163–64
    client names, this book, xv
    closing the circle, 205–8
    engagement, 126–27
    exercise tracking, 76–77
    final check-in, 208–11
    getting started, 52–54
    habits are hard to break, 103–4
    on High-Octane Brain role models,
        207–8

Meredith and Lou (*continued*)
  High-Octane Tracker completion, 206
  meeting each other, 34–36, 52
  MIND diet, 104–5
Mild cognitive impairment (MCI)
  Chandler, Dr. Melanie on, 231–39
  cognitive engagement and, 108
  defined, 14
  dementia versus, 15
  exercise and, 231, 235
  experience of living with, 15
  HABIT and, 15, 231, 232–33, 234–36,
    237–39
  Memory Support System and, 233–34
  mnemonic training and, 231–32
  statistics, 14
  stress and, 130
  treatment of, 15
MIND diet
  about, 83
  Alzheimer's and, 84
  benefits of, 99, 105, 106
  brain health and, 84
  challenges of integration, 90
  components, 86–89
  component services and scoring,
    100–101, 221, 223, 225, 228
  daily recommendations, 86
  Dr. Martha Clare Morris on, 89–92
  foods to limit, 87–88
  High-Octane Tracker, 99–102, 104
  integration of, 91
  recommendations, 83, 86–87
  research on, 85
  results of, 84–85
  saturated and trans fats and, 88
  servings in, 102
  tips for success, 101–2
  transition to, 102
  in U.S. Pointer clinical trial, 85
  vegetarians and, 87
  weekly recommendations, 86–87
Mindfulness
  acceptance and, 136, 137
  amplified High-Octane Brain benefits,
    135
  athletes, actors, and performers and,
    143
  awareness and, 136

awareness of joy and, 139
  benefits of, 133, 134, 146
  brain changes linked to, 141
  cognitive functioning and, 139–40, 141
  daily length of practice, 142–43
  defined, 134, 136
  depression and, 134–35, 141
  goal of, 138–39
  hippocampal growth and, 135, 140
  increased discomfort during, 138
  intentionality of, 137
  learning, 141–42
  meditation and prayer and, 136–37
  misconceptions about, 137
  negative thoughts and feelings and, 138
  settings where it's taught, 143–44
  sleep and, 160
  as stress management tool, 134–44, 149
Mindfulness-Based Cognitive Therapy, 142
Mindfulness-Based Stress Reduction, 141,
  142
Mind-set, 42–43, 55, 170
Mnemonic training, 231–32
Morris, Dr. Martha Clare, 81, 82, 89–92
Movement Matrix, 72
Multimodal Preventative Trail for
  Alzheimer's Disease (MIND-AD),
  14
Music therapy, 14

Name of someone you just met, forgetting,
  120–21
Navigational Forces
  about, 55–56
  brain health trajectories and, 45–48
  defined, 45
  foundational factors, 45–47
  health-related factors, 47
  lifestyle factors, 47–48
Neurogenesis, xi, 61
Neurons, 24–25, 61, 96, 155, 157
Neuroplasticity, 60–62
Neuroscience, xii
Neurotransmitters, 97
New information, forgetting, 123
Normal aging, 10, 11, 12
Nun Study, 20–22
Nutrients, 96–98, 106

Obesity, 47
Objects, misplacing, 121–22
OCTANE (One Change at a Time
    Accomplished Now equals
    Excellence), 77, 80, 206
Optimal brain aging, 26

Physical activity. *See* exercise
Plaques, 12, 13, 98
P-L-R method, 120, 121, 122, 123, 128. *See
    also* brain blips
Positive feedback loops, 48
Positive stress management strategies, 145,
    146, 149
Prayer, 136–37
PREDIMED, 82
Proactive interference, 140
Psychology Today blog, xii
PTSD (post-traumatic stress disorder), 141

Religion and spirituality, 14
REM (rapid eye movement) sleep, 152,
    153, 165
Resilience
    in action, 146, 218
    challenging notions of, 22
    recognizing, 146, 149
    as stress management tool, 144–45, 149
    SuperAgers and, 24, 25, 26
Resistance training, 69
Rey Auditory Verbal Learning Test, 23
Role models. *See* High-Octane Brain role
    models
Rush Memory and Aging Project, 22

Sabbagh, Dr. Marwan, 42–44, 92
Schwann, Theodor, 61
Shrinkage, brain, 11
Sister Bernadette, 21, 22
Sister Mary, 21–22
Sister Matthias, 21, 22
Sleep
    Alzheimer's and, 153–59, 165
    Alzheimer's-related cellular changes
        and, 154–56
    best practices, 159, 165
    cognitive functioning and, 153–59, 165
    cognitive symptoms and, 153
    deprivation, 150, 151, 158

exercise and, 159, 161
High-Octane Action Plan, 162
High-Octane Tracker, 163
importance of, 154
improving, 158, 160–62
memory processing and, 152–53
mindfulness and, 160
needs, 157, 165
problems, recognizing and treating,
    159–60
quality, improving, 157–59, 160–62
REM (rapid eye movement), 152, 153,
    165
research challenges, 158
schedule, following, 161
stages of, 152, 165
SWS (slow-wave sleep), 152, 153, 156,
    165
synergy of, 162
Takeaways, 165
tiredness and, 150–51
volunteering and, 160
Sleep apnea, 47
Sleep hygiene, 159, 165
Sleep medications, 160
Sleep-wake cycle, 154–55
Smoking, 47, 59
Social engagement, 24–25, 26, 114–15, 125
Social networks, 113
Spiritual fitness, 144, 149
Stern, Dr. Yaakov, 110–16
Stress
    about, 129–31
    Alzheimer's and, 129, 149
    depression and, 131, 132, 149
    high perceived, 130
    mild cognitive impairment (MCI) and,
        130
    questions measuring, 129–30
    studies of dementia and, 130–31
    SuperAgers and, 24
    treatment of, 132
Stress management
    flow and, 144
    High-Octane Action Plan, 145–46
    High-Octane Tracker, 146–47
    mindfulness and, 133–44, 149
    physical exercise and, 133–35
    positive strategies, 145, 146, 149

Stress management (*continued*)
    resilience and, 144–45, 146
    spiritual fitness and, 144, 149
    Takeaways, 149
    tools, 144–45
Sue, age 83 (role model), 184–87
SuperAgers
    about, 22
    classification of, 23
    commonalities of, 24–25
    concept of, 23
    defined, 22
    insights provided by, 28
    overview of, 26
    research findings, 24
    stress and, 24
    traits, cultivation of, 25
    Weintraub on, 22–24
Supplements, brain, 42, 43, 92–94, 105
Swedish women exercise study, 58–59
SWS (slow-wave sleep), 152, 153, 156, 165
Synonyms, substituting, 124–25

Tai chi, 15, 68, 69, 114, 234
Tangles, 12, 13
Tau, 156, 157

Three-Path Choice, 51, 53–54, 55, 56, 148, 206
Time, building brain health and, 44
Tip-of-the-tongue phenomenon, 124–25

Useful Field of View cognitive training, 119
U.S. POINTER clinical trial, 85

Vascular risk factors, 47
Vegetables, 83, 84, 86, 105
Vipassana retreats, 141
Virgil, age 53 (role model), 173–76
Volunteering, 160

Weintraub, Dr. Sandra, 22–24
WHO Guidelines, 50
Whole grains, 83, 86, 101
Whys, 38–39, 40, 52, 55, 126, 148, 206
Wine, brain health and, 83, 86, 94
Word-finding difficulties, 124–25
Working memory, 139, 140
Workup, 30
World wide FINGERS, 85

Yoga, 15, 68, 69, 142, 234

Picture Credits

Original High-Octane Tracker diagram design by Robert Johnson:
78, 219, 220, 222, 224, 227

Michelle Braun: 180, 189, 193, 197

Courtesy of Amy Friday: 169

Courtesy of Virgil Hammond: 173

KrPhotogs Photography: 176

Karen Postal: 184

Shutterstock.com: Cherstva: 124 (woman); danjazzia: 122 (keys); Leremy: 122 (figure 1), 124 (figures); Mr. Rashad: 51; Nadiinko: 122 (key ring); nelena: throughout (though bubble); NeMaria: throughout (arrow); Nizwa Design: cover, 1, 7, 57, 167; north100: 121 (figures, thinker), 122 (figure 2, thinker); RedKoala: 124 (lemon); vectomaker studio: 121 (bird)

Chris Solberg: 200

Vectorstock: Sileskyi: throughout (brain on tracker)

About the Author and Foreword Author

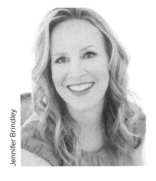

Jennifer Brindley

Dr. Michelle Braun is a Harvard- and Yale-trained board-certified neuropsychologist and a national leader in the field of brain health and cognitive functioning. She is a former instructor of psychiatry at Harvard Medical School and Assistant Director of Inpatient Mental Health at the Boston Veterans' Administration Hospital. In 2013, she was the featured presenter in a live 90-minute PBS *Next Avenue* television program on brain health. She has been interviewed as a brain health expert on Fox morning news, CBS, and iHeart Radio, and her work has been featured in national media outlets such as *Family Circle*, *Medical Daily*, HealthNewsDigest.com, and multiple newspapers. Her popular blog on brain health in *Psychology Today* has more than 200,000 views, and she has been an invited speaker for the Alzheimer's Association for the past 14 years.

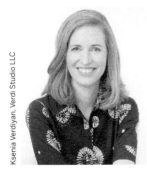

Ksenia Verdiyan, Verdi Studio LLC

Dr. Karen Postal is a past president of the American Academy of Clinical Neuropsychology and is a clinical instructor at Harvard Medical School. Her research focuses on improving communication about neuroscience with patients and the general public. She is the author of *Feedback That Sticks: The Art of Communicating Neuropsychological Assessment Results* and most recently, *Testimony That Sticks: The Art of Communicating Psychology and Neuropsychology to Jurors*. Dr. Postal has a private practice dedicated to helping people think better in school, at work, and throughout later life and a *Psychology Today* blog, *Think Better: Neuroscience for Everyday Life*.